THE LONG WAY HOME

The Long Way Home

How I Won the 1,000 Mile Iditarod Footrace with Persistence, Patience, and Passion

PETE RIPMASTER

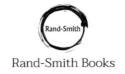

Rand-Smith Books

Rand-Smith Books
www.Rand-Smith.com

First Printing, 2021

Contents

Prologue

After reaching Rainy Pass and carefully navigating the dangerous Dalzell Gorge, I was excited to finally reach the mighty Tatina River. It was so beautiful that I had to stop and take it all in. I also had to remind myself how challenging it could be to cross a frozen, wild river.

That's what adventure is all about for me — living in the moment, remembering to be fully present. That's why I've spent most of my adult life challenging myself in the great outdoors. Setting audacious goals and crushing them has given me the inner peace that I desperately sought growing up.

Being from an affluent family, I was expected to be not only grateful but *fulfilled*. That's where I always got hung up. It took a long time for me to find the missing piece of the puzzle. I was not fulfilled. My soul was restless. I was certainly grateful for my fortuitous life circumstances, but it was obvious to me that I didn't fit in. None of it felt natural. I not only wanted something different, but I also desperately needed it. My path to fulfillment was arduous, to say the least. I battled demons at an early age when I experienced elementary school bullying on an epic scale. I don't care how self-confident you think you are: that shit changes you. It's a mental scar I've carried with me every day of my life.

Having the entire fifth grade class turn on me sent my younger self into a mental tailspin that left me with regular thoughts of ending the torture once and for all. Fortunately, with my parents' help, the situation was eventually resolved. In later years, I excelled in school sports which made my family proud and increased my popularity among my peers, but the damage was done. Partying my way through high school and college helped numb the pain and restlessness that had taken hold of my heart, but it did nothing to address the underlying issues. While the self-induced highs helped to tamp down the demons, I continued to make poor life choices as I bounced from one college to the next in search of a place where I felt whole.

Through trial and error, I found that testing my physical and mental limits through ultrarunning gave me exactly what I had been searching for all those years. The process of identifying a challenge, researching it, obsessing over it, training for it, and finally conquering it, satisfied every part of my soul. The aches and pains that lingered in my body for days, weeks, and even months afterward brought a smile to my face because they were a physical reminder of the spiritual nirvana I had attained. That sweet satisfaction fed my spirit and filled me with a completeness that reminded me of how fortunate I was in my everyday life. But then, it's just a matter of time before those aches subside, and my body longs for another far-flung adventure.

In 2013, I serendipitously found out that the world-famous Iditarod Trail could be done during winter, on foot, without dogs. Hallelujah! I knew I had found my adventure destiny. The human-powered Iditarod Trail Invitational (ITI) began a week before the famous dog sled race. Annually, since 1997, adventure athletes have chosen to bike, hike, or ski the historic trail for 350 miles from the town of Knik over the Alaska Range to McGrath. In 2000, athletes who completed the 350-mile race were then eligible to register for the ultimate 1,000-mile challenge to Nome the following year. The name was officially changed to the ITI in 2002.

I had grown up in Michigan reading books like *Hatchet, Endurance,* and *The Call of the Wild,* so "last frontier" stories always held a special place in my heart. However, none of those stories affected me quite like the story of Balto, which spoke to the beginnings of the Iditarod. In fact, I made a promise to myself in 5th grade that I would one day chase my own Iditarod dreams. In the early 2000s, I got the opportunity to work for Iditarod mushers in Alaska while I was grieving my mom's loss to breast cancer. With the help of talented mentors and a healthy dose of hard work, I became familiar with the rugged terrain, wild animals, and unpredictable weather of Alaska. I knew then, from a place deep down in my soul, that this race would be the ultimate adventure. Completing the 350-mile portion was very tough, but I conquered it, twice.

However, when I attempted that 1,000-mile race, I quickly realized I was up against the most grueling challenge of my life—not to mention that damn Tatina River.

Chapter One

The Beginning

Somewhere, there's a picture of me when I was about two years old with a Detroit Tigers hat perched on my big fat head, a baseball in one hand and a bat in the other. I was born in November of 1976 in Ann Arbor, Michigan, as the first son in my family. Dad loved sports. Both he and my grandfather played football for Michigan State, so I suppose athletics was part of my genetic makeup. My mother was also a phenomenal athlete who didn't fancy losing. Fortunately, I took to sports easily, a natural no matter the game. It wasn't long before I began to get attention from teachers, coaches, and family friends commenting on the way I swung a bat or ran a ball down the field.

At first, those accolades were a little unnerving. Sports came so easily to me that I didn't understand what the fuss was about. It wasn't like I worked really hard or focused on winning; I was having fun. The game wasn't as important to me as just being active and staying busy. Because of that, it felt like a healthy, happy childhood. We had the white picket fence and the nice house, but sometimes I got the uneasy feeling that things were almost too good, almost too easy.

I clearly remember one of my first acts of rebellion. Photos. Family pictures. To me, they were sheer torture. When I see a

1

picture of myself as a little kid, I look at the nice, expensive clothes and the neatly combed hair and think, "Who is that?" That's not me. That was never me. What I remember is everything that happened behind the scenes. My mother saying for the millionth time, "Comb your hair." "Put on your sweater." "Sit still and smile." "Act like a good little boy ." I just could not understand why she would want a picture of me that looked so unlike the real me.

When I was in elementary school, I started to realize that not everyone lived the way we did. Talking about money and finances was always vague in our house. Mom would come up to me and say, "Peter, here's a $10,000 check that came in the mail for you from Grandma and Grandpa Dobson."

"Great, Mom. Wow!"

"No, you just need to sign it. Then it goes in the bank."

"But—"

"We put it into a fund. It's for tax purposes, honey. Don't think about it."

On my mom's side of the family, my Grandpa Dobson was a great businessman, and my Grandma Dobson inherited a valuable stock portfolio from her parents. So, the two of them together did very well financially. My dad's parents were more blue-collar and made it a point to live life to the absolute fullest. When it came to my parents, they viewed money differently. Mom was humble, stubborn, and fiscally cautious. My dad was the opposite. His philosophy was that life was for living. Money was to be enjoyed. You can't take it with you! I'm sure their differing viewpoints caused more issues between them than I truly understood.

My father was also a very hard-working businessman and quite successful in his own right, but he would spend every damn dime he made, much to my mother's chagrin. I'm not sure of the best way to teach kids about money, but I know that was not it. It was confusing for me to get checks in the mail that I couldn't use while Dad was buying whatever the hell he wanted. There was no consistency, no financial education, and no explanation. It was the only life I knew.

After we moved to Birmingham, Michigan, things went to another level. It was the '80s, and the auto industry was booming. Everyone in our area had money, including my family. Million-dollar houses were the norm and, of course, that meant the nicest cars and priciest country clubs. For a lot of the kids I met, it was their mission in life to let everyone know how much money their family had. However, I never connected with that lifestyle, so I always felt like an outsider even though I tried to fit in as best as I could. And I wasn't the only one. My sister Sarah was born first, then me, and finally my brother Scott rounded out our family. I was always the crazy, certifiable middle child. Sarah and I were close when I was younger, but as we got older, she and her friends were pretty tough on me. I was already sensitive because I had a speech impediment that made pronouncing the letter "r" difficult, which made saying "Peter" difficult and frustrating. I'd pronounce it "Pee-do."

Kids have the cruel ability to zero in on weakness, and attack. When my sister and her friends would come to the house, they called me names and teased me. My usual tactic was to first go to my room, and if they followed me, I'd lock myself in the bathroom. I just needed some space to get away and clear my head. I hated that feeling of being belittled and bullied for something I couldn't control. It made me feel helpless and alone.

One time they started up and, as usual, I locked myself in the bathroom. That didn't seem to deter them, and they kept yelling from the other side of the door, "Pee-do! Poor Pee-do!" Then I heard Sarah saying it, too. That was the last straw. She knew how it made me feel, and she was encouraging them to gang up on me. I flung the door open and chased Sarah downstairs and into the kitchen. They circled me like a pack of wild dogs, and I went into survival mode. Sarah yelled "Pee-do" at me, and I snapped.

I grabbed her by the neck, somehow lifted her off the ground, and started slamming her head into the cupboard. It was like I had no control over my actions. The rage and pain and frustration took over. When I saw blood dripping down the cabinet, I let go of her, ran back upstairs, and locked myself in my bathroom again. I knew my dad was going to come home and whoop my ass. It is definitely a moment that I regretted then, and now, because it showed a side of me that I'd never experienced; but it also made me realize something. I'd always known that I had this feeling deep inside that, despite the nice life and the athletic success, I'd always felt a silent rage, an uneasiness that I couldn't identify.

In fifth grade, there was a certain loudmouth who other kids tended to gravitate to for some odd reason. One day he apparently came to the conclusion that he didn't like me. Since he commanded the attention of most of the class, he said anything and everything to make sure others didn't like me, either. The mob mentality very quickly evolved, and soon the entire class of eleven-year-olds was against me. I was no angel as a kid and caused more than my fair share of trouble, but I had never been a bully.

Even the kids whose parents were friends with my folks turned on me. I thought it would blow over, but it continued to escalate. It was nothing short of brutal. I was a pre-teen boy trying to figure out who I was, and every day I had to face a torrent of hate and anger at school. After already enduring tough episodes with my sister and her friends, I knew the detrimental effects bullying can have, and the fact that it was happening again was more than I thought I could bear.

Every day after school, I'd confide in my parents that I was being pushed on the playground, being spit at in the hallways, and dodging flying food in the cafeteria. I did not have a single ally, and I learned not to trust any classmates. The teachers didn't take any action, and there was no support from the administration, although it was obvious to everyone what was happening. This went on for almost an entire school year.

It didn't matter how good I had things at home or how many points I scored on the court; when I got to class, I was treated like a pariah. As the weeks and months passed, my mood became darker and darker. That uneasy feeling inside me began to take over. Sadness was all I could focus on. I turned inward, reading stories of extreme survival in harsh conditions. For some reason, they gave me hope. They kept the sadness at bay, if only temporarily. Anything about Alaska, nature, and animals resonated with me: stories where there were as few people as possible. That's around the time I discovered writers like Jack London and became obsessed with books like *The Call of the Wild, White Fang,* and *To Build a Fire.*

My parents could tell I was in a bad place, and I finally felt safe enough to open up to them about my true feelings—that I wanted to end the misery and give in to the darkness. School was everything to me at 11 years old. It was my entire world, and everyone there was against me. Those fantastic tales in the books provided a much-needed escape for my mind, but once the story was over, the hopelessness fell back on me like an Alaskan avalanche. It was as if that torment increased every day, weighing me down, testing me to see how much I could handle. That's when I told them that I wanted to put an end to everything. I was done. I wasn't taking the easy way out, but after months of torture, I didn't want to go through another day. The darkness had consumed me, had robbed me of the carefree little boy I once was. My outgoing nature had been compromised; my spirit was broken.

When my parents grasped what I was telling them, they reacted. My mother was concerned, probably realizing that I was in a deep depression and that if I were sharing something so dark, I must have been seriously contemplating my next move. My father was much more direct in his approach. That night, he went to the house of the boy who had been most responsible for the bullying. Dad was a big, tough guy, not someone people wanted to mess with. Apparently, when the child's father answered the door, my dad asked to speak directly to his son. Soon the kid was outside, face-to-face with my father, who was poking the kid in the chest with his finger. "This is going to stop! You are not going to mess with my son anymore!"

The next day, I was even more apprehensive about going to school because I hadn't been with my dad the night before, so I didn't know what had actually happened. I braced myself for the worst, which was a good thing because all hell broke loose. The situation was exponentially more intense because I became the one who told a grownup what was happening. So now I was a baby and a tattletale, and that meant more torment.

I came home and said, "Dad, I can't deal with this. I can't. I'm trying to turn the other cheek and everything you've been telling me to do, but it's worse."

He said, "You know what, tomorrow when you go to school and someone pushes you, I want you to punch them right in their face."

"Yeah, right, Dad."

"Peter, I'm dead serious right now. I've had it. This is how we're going to take care of it."

So the next day, as usual, I had a group of kids around me on the playground, and I heard one of them say to another, "Hey, push Peter in the back. It will be funny." So I knew what was coming, and I just turned around and punched this kid right in the kisser, knocking him straight on his back. Then, I dropped to my knees and kept wailing on him. I pinned his arms and windmilled my fists until the principal ran out and yanked me off him. I'd had a year of anger built up, and I was like a wild animal.

As I sat in his office, the principal told me I was in "so much trouble" as he dialed the phone. "Mr. Ripmaster, your son is in deep trouble. You need to come and pick him up NOW!"

Not long after, Dad stormed into the office. Just as the principal launched into a rant of how I was such a bad kid, Dad cut him off. "You guys were not protecting my son, so I told him to defend himself. This is what happens when the administration does nothing about the intense bullying that has gone on for a year! Peter was working hard to not get physical, but he had no choice. I'm proud of my son for this." He put his arm around me and said, "We're going to go get an ice cream cone." You should've seen the looks on their faces!

Not even a day after the incident, I was inundated with phone calls from kids at school apologizing for how they had treated me and asking if we could now be friends. It was odd to see them all suddenly respect me and want to be my friend, but I welcomed it. I needed it. I was glad that the circumstances had changed, but I didn't think that I could trust any of them completely, or anybody for that matter. How could I? The damage had been done.

Fortunately, junior high was a much different experience. For many kids, middle school is like the ninth circle of hell. It's a time when puberty, hormones, and self-discovery are trapped in a self-contained ecosystem, and it can wreak havoc on self-esteem. I had just come out of the worst year of my life, and middle school meant a new beginning. It was as if a light switch had flipped. Suddenly, I was one of the best athletes in the school, playing point guard on the basketball team, pitching on my baseball team, and playing linebacker on the football field. I was just starting to get attention from pretty girls at school and things could not have been better.

It was a turning point for me in a good way, but it also gave me an interesting perspective on human nature and the pack mentality that can develop. I was well-known in school, but I kept my circle of friends small and carefully chosen. Even then, I didn't trust them with all my secrets. I was grateful that the negative thoughts had subsided, but any time I saw someone bullied or mercilessly teased, those feelings came flooding back. So my coping mechanism was to hold my cards close to the vest, shove the feelings down, and focus on the good things that were happening.

My relationship with my father was also growing and changing. In the summer of 1989, when I was 12, my dad, brother, and I went to colorful Colorado for the first time, my first real western boys' trip. Dad's best friend from Michigan State had a rustic 4,500-acre ranch outside of Telluride. The four of us went into a mercantile in the town of Ridgway on our way to Telluride. I looked up at the magazine rack, and it was like my hormones exploded. There was a *Playboy* with Pamela Anderson on the cover wearing an unbuttoned boarding-school type jacket. She was in all her blonde glory, and I was mesmerized. I turned to my dad, this cowboy tough guy, and said, "I need that! Will you buy it for me?"

He said, "I don't know if I'm ready to do that, Pete. First, I think you kind of have to prove yourself out here in the west."

"Dad, I'll do A-N-Y-T-H-I-N-G!"

"Ok, how about this? If you drink a shot of Jack Daniel's around the fire tonight, I'll buy you a *Playboy*."

When we were sitting around the campfire with a bunch of cowboys, I took the shot glass and slammed the whiskey down in one gulp. The brown liquor burned my throat like nothing I'd ever known, and the guys got a good laugh at my reaction. Then Dad reached around and pulled out a plastic-covered *Playboy* magazine. Back then, Telluride had a different feel. It was a western town, totally cowboy-focused, and

I gravitated toward that. At the ranch outside of town, there was even more of a cowboy culture, and I saw a world that was much different from the cookie-cutter houses that lined the streets in our well-manicured suburban neighborhood.

Every weekend, those cowboys would bring the money they earned that week to the little bunkhouse on the property to drink, gamble, and shoot pool . I'd watch my dad hustle them in pool as they laughed, drank, and shared stories that I didn't fully understand. After the game, they'd talk about kicking my dad's ass because he cleaned them out. Dad would just laugh. "It's your fault because you suck at pool. Try harder next time!" It was an exciting time for me, and the freedom and camaraderie fed my twelve-year-old soul. It was like I'd found what had been missing. I loved it all, whether I was watching a cowboy check a cow to verify its pregnancy or sitting around the campfire listening to Merle Haggard songs played on beat-up guitars. This couldn't have been more different than Birmingham, Michigan, where kids I knew were bragging about Polo shirts and fancy overseas trips.

Maybe my simpler outlook came from my Grandma Dobson . She was always very conservative and cautious with her inheritance. Blame it on her Scottish blood, but that's probably why she and my grandfather were so prosperous. She was born in 1915 and went through the Great Depression, and that made an impact on her and many from that generation. Money was to be respected and protected. Her family moved to the Ann Arbor area in 1936 and she became a Michigander through and through.

She and my mom had a close relationship even after we moved to Birmingham for Dad's job. I didn't see her as often, but she was always supportive of my school activities and sporting events. And her values never wavered.

My adolescence was filled with a sense of yearning and searching. The Colorado trip opened my eyes to a different world, a more rustic place that resonated with me. Despite excelling in sports back in Birmingham, I never felt truly fulfilled. I played tennis in middle school and traveled to tournaments, practicing five days a week. It consumed me until it didn't. I got burned out and just stopped. Trying my hand at different sports helped keep me distracted and busy.

After tennis, I turned my focus to golf. One time, Dad took me to play in a father-son golf tournament at Red Run Golf Club in Royal Oak, Michigan. During the closest-to-the-pin contest, I watched Chuck Kocsis, a Michigan PGA champion, put that little white ball about five feet from the pin, and the crowd roared. I walked up to the officials and said, "I want to hit a ball, too. I want to be in this contest." I think they were humoring me when they allowed me to give it a try. I took out my driver, gave the ball a solid whack, and the crowd watched as it soared 150 yards down the fairway and came to a stop on the green, right beside Chuck's ball. Chuck was a good sport and shouted to the crowd, "Give the kid the trophy!"

The same happened with soccer. I took to it easily and was quickly recognized as a valuable team member. During one game, I scored five or six goals during the first half. Then my coach said, "Pete, I'm going to have to take you out of the game. You're not going to play in the second half." As soon as I was out of the game, our opponents scored a couple of quick goals. Later in the game, the score was tied, and the coach yelled, "Ok, Pete, I'm putting you back in." I scored the winning goal, and everyone went nuts. I could see how much joy the win gave them, but it never did much for me.

I probably could have pursued a professional career in tennis, soccer, or golf if I'd had the focus, and most importantly, the desire. For some reason, shifting my attention helped keep my mind busy so I wasn't alone with my thoughts. High school meant playing football, basketball, baseball—it didn't really matter to me. I was all-state in multiple sports and recruited by several colleges. One of the last football games I played during high school took place at the Pontiac Silverdome where the Detroit Lions played. I caught a touchdown pass that helped win the game. Then for my last baseball game, I was invited to the Michigan All-Star game at the old Detroit Tiger Stadium. I hit an RBI single that also helped win the game. Precious memories.

Despite being gifted with this innate athletic ability, it never felt comfortable for me. I didn't want to be lumped in with the football players and that mob-like mentality. Some saw it as teamwork and dedication, but to me it was dangerous. I'd seen firsthand how destructive those situations could become. Still, I felt pressured by my father and my coaches to excel. An All-American at our school had gone on to play quarterback at Northwestern, and he was the pride of our community. So, there was a hope that I'd pick up that baton and run with it. I knew that was the end goal, and I wanted to make everyone happy, so I tried. I learned the plays, went all out at every practice, and found success on the field. It was later when I was showered with attention that I immediately pulled back. Being under that magnifying glass made me feel incredibly uncomfortable. After a lifetime of protecting my inner thoughts and fears, I felt exposed and unprotected. It made me uneasy, and I knew that I couldn't play that role the way everyone had hoped I would.

However, my coach was not giving up on me so easily. He pulled me aside one day and said, "Peter, it's obvious. You don't want to play quarterback at all. That's where I think you belong, but it's up to you. I don't want to lose you. Is there another position you'd rather play?"

"How about linebacker or tight end?"

Done. I know it was a disappointment for my dad because he got a charge out of telling his buddies, "My boy is a quarterback, and he's on his way to Michigan State." I give him credit because even though he didn't want me to change positions, he was always in the stands cheering me on. The pivotal game was during my junior year: a playoff game against Brother Rice, a highly ranked private school. When that team entered the field, our coach worried about our lives but never gave up the belief that we had a chance. It was a true David and Goliath scenario. My dad and Grandpa Rip were in the stadium watching every move I made. As they got drunk on schnapps that they'd smuggled in their jackets, we eked out a 14-13 win. This win is still considered one of the biggest upsets in Michigan high school football history.

Looking back, I cannot help but wonder what would have happened if I had pursued any of those opportunities, if I had taken advantage of my athletic abilities. The truth is that I'd always had that inherent feeling of not belonging, of feeling alone, of being surrounded by inescapable sadness. Somehow, my classmates were able to detect that weakness and capitalize on it. The incessant bullying had turned me even more inward and more wary of getting close to others. Throwing myself into sports should have been the way out. In theory, it should have given me structure, confidence, reassurance, popularity—and it did do all those things, but it never felt right.

In fact, it had the opposite effect on me. Where I should have been enjoying the attention, I was retreating because it made me stressed and anxious. The more I was celebrated for my achievements, the heavier the blanket of depression felt. In the beginning, I thought everyone wore a mask of happiness in public to hide the dark, shameful secrets that bubbled just beneath the surface.

I tried to fit in at first. I hung out with my teammates and worked to build the camaraderie that I knew was necessary for a cohesive team, but it was always a struggle for me. Once, our JV football team was playing Hazel Park, a less-affluent area filled with hard-working blue-collar families. Some of the guys on their team already had full beards. They were a sturdy bunch for sure.

One of the guys on our team decided it would be funny to draw dollar signs across our helmets as an intimidation tactic and a nod to our economic status. I was so disgusted by it that I refused to take part, which of course was a red flag from a team perspective. There was no tolerance for anything except complete dedication, and after my experiences in fifth grade, that didn't work for me.

My earlier social interactions gave me a different perspective and made me question things instead of giving in to blind acceptance. Within my family, I was able to confide in my mother and my grandmother, and I accepted and loved my father for the man he was. Yet even at home, I never completely felt at ease. I always had my guard up, never putting my defenses down for anyone. It was my only protection from a world that I'd learned could be cruel, especially toward someone who didn't follow social norms and do what was expected.

Living in a wealthy area didn't help either because I was expected to embrace the material things that surrounded all of us. A lot of my friends saw that as an extension of themselves and anyone who didn't do the same was the odd man out. I'm not going to say I didn't like those things, but they didn't define me or consume me. If I even dared mention the peaceful expanse of Colorado or the tranquil beauty of Alaska, I was met with blank stares as if I would be crazy to want anything other than what I had. It was yet another example of my inability to assimilate and go with the flow.

I'm not sure why camaraderie didn't come to me as naturally as athletics did, but it was a fact. The distraction of sports had provided a temporary reprieve from the depths of my own mind, but it was becoming less and less effective. Then, in my sophomore year of high school, I found another way to not only suppress the negative thoughts but escape them altogether. That method was effective because it didn't just distract me; it altered my mind and allowed me to create a world that I could fill with things that made me happy. Sure, it was only in my mind, and it was only temporary; but if I kept it up, maybe it would become my reality. Chasing that dragon quickly consumed me, but I felt it was my only chance to survive in a world where I felt like I didn't belong.

The drinking, pot use, and drugs not only affected my relationships, my family, and my athletic ability; they almost killed me.

Chapter Two

Dr. Jekyll

When it became time for me to get a car as I was getting close to 16, the plan was for me to get my sister's hand-me-down Eagle Talon. It was a small sports car with a stick shift, and I had absolutely no idea how to drive it. One day, my dad took me to an empty parking lot and attempted to teach me how to drive a manual transmission. It did not go well at all. He would drive while explaining how to engage the clutch and shift gears. It looked pretty easy. When he finally let me try, I found it to be much more difficult than it looked. I was terrible at it and would lurch and stall every time I tried to switch gears. I just couldn't figure out the timing of letting go of the clutch while starting to gently press the gas. My dad was getting seriously frustrated every time I stalled out. After about an hour with no progress, we had both had it. I remember my dad saying, "I can't believe you can hit home runs, knock down three-pointers, and score touchdowns, but you can't figure out how to drive a Goddamn stick!" That sent me over the edge. I said, "I don't like this tiny piece of shit anyway, why the hell don't you just trade it in for an old truck for me?" I guess he understood my frustrations.

We hastily decided on a used, AUTOMATIC Chevy Blazer, and I couldn't have been happier. The very first night I had it, I drove my girlfriend and a few other friends to a friend's house to party a bit. After we left the house, my girlfriend, who was new to drinking, puked all over the inside and outside of the vehicle after one too many beers. When I think about it now, that pretty much summed up my high school years. I was *never* an angel and always felt like a misfit, giving in to every teenage temptation I could find. I was smoking weed daily, trying mind-altering drugs, and hiding empty 40s on my bookshelf behind worn copies of *My Side of the Mountain* and James Michener's *Alaska*.

My sister was a senior when I was a first-year student, and I didn't like being known as her little brother. I wanted to be my own man, so I tried hard to establish an identity that was all mine. A bonfire out in a field, a concert in a nearby town; if there was an opportunity to party, I was there. Some of my friends would pile in a car and we'd drive to Canada via the Ambassador Bridge. It was kind of cool that after a short drive we could be in a different country. One night, we ended up getting into a fight with some skinheads at a bar in Windsor. We drove back in bloody silence. The next morning, my sister walked into the laundry room as I was tossing my clothes in the washer.

"Jesus, Peter, what the hell happened?"

"I got into a little fight, I guess."

"I really don't know who you are anymore."

She was right. I was spiraling and there was no stopping me. The warning signs were there. She and my mother pointed them out, but I was as stubborn as a country mule. Somehow, I justified my high school behavior by excelling in sports. It wouldn't have been uncommon for me to star in a baseball game before going off to a Grateful Dead concert and consuming a small handful of mind-altering mushrooms.

Coaches and teachers were certainly aware of my antics, but it was written off as sowing my wild oats. I got a pass because I was winning on the field and on the court.

In my junior year, I played football in the fall and as soon as I turned in my pads for the season, I jumped into basketball practice. One day, one of the star players on the basketball team was in the locker room getting taped up when he said, "Pete, I saw you got a recruiting letter in the mail for football."

"Shut up, man." I figured he was egging me on because I was on his turf. Typical high school stuff. I wasn't buying it. "Who's it from?"

"Notre Dame. Pete, I'm not kidding. Go downstairs and look on the table."

I went down there and sure enough, there was a letter on fancy cardstock with a golden football helmet logo at the top left. The letter was from Notre Dame and said they were officially recruiting me for football. I thought it was a joke. My coach had always told me I was really good, but I wasn't one of those who ate, slept, and crapped football. It just wasn't in my blood. A few weeks later, I was walking down the hallway with some of the art crowd who I hung out with when I was away from sports. I had on my skater pants with the wide legs and checkered Vans on my feet. A friend stopped me in the hallway and said, "There's a Notre Dame coach in the football office talking about you." Apparently, my coach had filled the guy in on my extracurricular partying activities and said I probably was not what they were looking for in South Bend.

I guess Lou Holtz, Notre Dame's head coach at the time, was set on seeing more of me though because I was invited as a recruit to their annual spring game. My dad, my best friend Smoke, and I went to South Bend, Indiana, to check it out. When I got there, I saw recruits out on the field and quarterback Ron Powlus on the sidelines signing autographs for eager fans. I made my way onto the field and over to the sidelines. I went over and started talking to the quarterback about recruitment. Then, one of the fans asked for my autograph. I assured him that I was just a recruit and that he didn't want it, but he was persistent. "A lot of recruits come in and play good ball. Then it's harder to get autographs." So Powlus would sign a ball and then pass it to his left for me to sign. That went on for a while as Dad and my buddy laughed from the stands. Just as I was about to step away, another little kid approached, so I signed one more ball. Then I saw him take it to his dad who looked at me and then my signature and said, "Who the hell is Peter Ripmaster?"

It was exactly the reminder I needed to keep me in check. I'd had several Division II and III teams reach out about recruitment, but I'd gotten it in my head that I was too good for them. People said my hands were like glue because I could catch any pass that was thrown to me. That was my skill. But based on my lackluster dedication to the game, a Division II or Division III team was probably where I rightfully belonged. A Division I team wasn't going to sign me to play football because of my lack of size and speed. The last game I played in high school football was at the Pontiac Silverdome. I caught a touchdown pass that game, and that's how I said "so long" to that sport.

In my senior year after football, I switched to baseball and didn't have a great year. While I got plenty of RBIs and home runs, I struck out a lot and didn't have the average I'd had my junior year. Shit, I didn't even win team MVP. Somehow, I was still invited to play in the prestigious Michigan All-Star game at Tiger Stadium. I thought of my selection as lucky because of the way I had played. Still, I went to the game to give it a shot with my family and friends cheering me on from the stands. During the game, I waited in the dugout and watched as one by one our guys struck out. Later in the game, I hadn't had a chance to play at all, but the coach said, "We'll certainly give you a shot at bat."

I was psyched because I still wanted to do my best and make my family proud even if I wasn't the best athlete on the field. I swore I could hear my dad's voice as I sidled up to the plate. The pitcher was a huge guy, a real powerhouse, and his first pitch was pure smoke. The pitcher's mound was much higher than I was used to, which threw off my perception. The ball zoomed by and slapped the catcher's mitt with a thud as the umpire yelled, "Strike!" I shot the umpire a glance and said, "Are you kidding me? That almost hit the plate!"

"It was right down the middle, son. Strike one!"

So I got ready for the next pitch, ready to make contact. Then before I knew it, the ball had whizzed by again.

"Strike two!"

This time I heard my dad yell from the stands, "Swing the damn bat, Peter!"

As I stepped out of the batter's box for a quick second, I told myself to slow down and think it through. The pitcher probably assumed I was some star struck wannabe who didn't know what he was doing. I figured since his first two pitches had been strikes, he wasn't going to waste his time with a pitch out of the strike zone, which would've been normal with a 0-2 count. I needed to be ready for another fastball. I figured whatever was going to happen, I needed to go out swinging, no matter what. Then it came, the third fastball in a row, and this time I connected, hitting a laser of a line drive right into the gap behind second base. My teammate on second base scored and I was rewarded with an important RBI single. I was on first base where a legendary coach patted me on the back as my dad was going nuts in the stands. That was my only at-bat of the game, and I made the most of it.

The rush of adrenaline that came from those moments in sports was what made it worthwhile until I pushed harder into the party scene. My parents dealt with my escapades in different ways. Being the tough guy, my dad held tight to the old-school mentality of machismo and bravado. After my issues in elementary school, he was proud to see his boy following in his footsteps, both on and off the field, and the partying was absolutely excused. Boys will be boys. I had much more of an emotional connection with my mom, but neither of my parents had put an emphasis on education until my junior year. By then, it was too little, way too late.

One day my mom came to me and said, "Your grade point average isn't great, and I'm worried that you're going to have trouble getting into a good school. Why don't you work hard to prepare for taking the ACT?"

She enrolled me in one of those catch-up classes where they try to make up for years of academic indifference by cramming targeted information into resistant teen brains. Once I got in there, I knew it was a colossal waste of time. There was just no way I'd be able to learn everything I needed to know to take the ACT, and the worst part was I didn't really care. I just saw it as a hassle. On the day of the ACT test, the proctor distributed five versions to ensure honesty, but I noticed that the girl in the row next to me had the same version I had. She looked pretty damn smart, too! As she methodically worked her way through each question, I shot a glance over and followed her lead. I was so calculated that I purposefully included a few different answers to mask the deception.

A few weeks later, I was with a best friend in West Virginia doing some whitewater rafting. While I was there, my mother called me one night and told me, "ALL of that hard work you put in paid off! Your ACT score was incredible, Peter! I'm so proud of you!" My usual school grades were B's or more likely C's, but my unexpected ACT results weren't questioned in the slightest. I fooled them all and wasn't about to correct anybody's misconceptions. There were certain expectations of me, and I went along with them. At that point, I didn't even care. I was completely selfish and had zero remorse. It's not a point in my life that I'm proud of, but I can't pretend it didn't happen, either. There were things that happened during that time that will always profoundly affect me. Things that are far too personal to write about, heavy.

When I experimented with alcohol and mind-altering drugs, it was a way to suppress my inner thoughts and escape a world where I didn't feel that I belonged. I graduated from alcohol and pot and didn't want to stop there. I had a couple of very scary LSD trips that should have scared me straight, but I was determined to keep exploring, especially if sports weren't going to be my thing. After one of those bad trips my senior year, I somehow made it home to find my mom sobbing on the sofa. I was going to college a couple of days later, and she had gone through some of my "hidden" dresser drawers. Of course, she'd found my drug paraphernalia and a stack of *Penthouse* magazines, among other things a teenage boy would never want his mother to see. It hit her hard. I'm sure she'd had her suspicions, but when they were confirmed, it was just too much for her to bear. I had just come home from a wild night, and she was practically having a breakdown. It was an intense scene.

Finally, she managed to say, "You are not going to college. You're going to rehab."

I tried to calm her down. "Mom, it's just teenage stuff. No big deal. There's no way I'm going to rehab. I'm fine." Plans had already been set for my folks to drop me off at the frat house I was moving into at the University of Kansas, and now she was having second thoughts.

"You absolutely need to take a year off," she said, "and get yourself together."

"No, Mom. It's not that serious. This is how I roll." To top it off, she wanted to take me out to the store to buy some supplies and clothes for college, but I had made plans to party with my friends. "Mom, I don't care about new clothes. I have clothes. I don't need anything." I'd never heard a bad word come out of her mouth, but she'd had it with me.

"Goddamn it, Peter! I'm trying to do nice things for you, and you don't even fucking appreciate it!"

I was knee-deep into my ridiculous punkish phase, so no one could get through to me. "Now you're going to cuss me out, Mom? Is that where we're at?" I think of that behavior now and it absolutely crushes me.

We all know hindsight is 20/20, but if I had taken advantage of those sports opportunities, who knows what could have happened. When I saw teammates getting heavily recruited, it pissed me off because I felt like I'd deserved it more than they did; but of course, I was delusional. Most of those guys focused on their health, worked out constantly, and practiced daily. Here I was, coasting by on God-given talent without fully realizing my potential. I was just a punk who was stressing the hell out of his parents and coaches.

Substance abuse, partying, and putting myself in dangerous situations were effective ways of keeping my mind distracted. I was able to push back the bad thoughts. At the first tinge of that ominous wave of sadness, I'd grab a 40 or a joint and jump in my car, anything to stave off the inevitable. Depression was an illness that my father suffered from as well. There were times, I would come to find out later, when he'd spend the entire day in bed, and not leave the house for days. I didn't understand what was going on, but those crippling episodes must have been a blow to his ego. He was never one to admit weakness and would fall into a cycle of frustration and despair.

I know I put my parents through hell, and I should have communicated my desire to explore nature and learn more about life outside of our posh community. When I took an environmental studies class during my senior year, the teacher pulled me aside and said, "You know, I can tell that this is something that interests you." She was right. She saw something in me that I was not confident enough to explore at the time. I was too busy being the rebel of the family, causing havoc to hide the fact that I just didn't fit in.

The truth is, at that time, I didn't feel comfortable in my own skin. Birmingham, Michigan, was a great, safe town to grow up in, but I had a heavy feeling that most people didn't live the way I did. My early trip to Telluride, Colorado, showed me that there was a big, wild world out there, and I wanted to leave my own mark on it. Rather than go to Michigan State like my grandpa, grandma, dad, mom, and sister, I wanted to rock the boat, and it was high time for me to get the hell out of Michigan. One of the first schools I was accepted to was KU in Lawrence, Kansas, and I fell in love with it the first time I visited. It seemed like a perfect place to blaze my own path, and that's exactly what I did. I longed for freedom and pretty girls. Lawrence didn't disappoint!

Chapter Three

Lost & Found

I was looking for a college to attend in 1994. My parents had dear friends from their alma mater, Michigan State, with a son who was at the University of Kansas. I was intrigued by KU and accepted there, probably only because of my ACT score. Nonetheless, Mom called the friends and said, "Hey, can I have your son's number? You know, I'd love for Pete to connect with him and see what the living situation is like there." So, I called the guy, and he was super nice.

Toward the end of our talk, he said, "You need to come check out our frat house."

I thought, *hell* no. I had already been to several frat parties with my older friends up at Michigan State and that was most certainly not me. I said, "No, thank you. Thanks for asking though."

We talked a bit more and he said, "Just come down to Lawrence this summer. I'll pick you up and introduce you to a bunch of the guys. You can see what they're all about and if you like it, great, but if you don't, no worries."

Mom agreed, "You should do it, Peter."

When I got there, he picked me up as promised. The first night, I ended up getting rip-roaring drunk. My new friends had been really nice to me, but by the next morning, I thought I had probably screwed it up by getting so hammered. To my surprise, they asked me to join the fraternity. They were a fun group of guys and we all got along, so despite my reservations about Greek life, I decided to go for it.

At the beginning of the fall semester, several cars pulled up to the frat house as parents dropped off their sons for the adventure of a lifetime. My parents drove me down to Lawrence and ended up staying in town overnight before their drive back to Michigan.

"We'll come pick you up tomorrow morning for breakfast, and then we'll say goodbye," Mom called out the window as Dad pulled away from the curb.

The other guys were loaded down with grooming products and designer wear. Then there was me, with a few clothes, deodorant, skateboard, bong, and toothpaste. That was it. I was definitely out of my element. The minute I stepped in the house and all the parents were out of sight, I found myself in a pledge line with 31 other guys. "OK, get into two rows of 16, you little shits! First guy goes to the keg and fills up, then goes to the back of the line to chug his beer before getting to the front of the line again. You pieces of crap need to empty these kegs fast!"

As we set out to empty our kegs as instructed, the upperclass students started yelling and throwing things at us. I jumped in like a trooper and did my part to drink that cheap beer as quickly as possible. Somewhere in the middle of the craziness, I realized I'd been sucked into a hazing scenario that I'd promised myself I'd never allow. After the treatment I'd received in elementary school, I couldn't believe it was happening. Not only that, but I'd also chosen this scenario, voluntarily! These guys had seemed so cool at first; then I was being yelled at like I was subhuman.

As pledges, we were called frogs. "You fucking frogs! Drink! Drink!" Maybe I was naive, but I had no idea it was going to be like that. I'd been coasting along just fine in high school and thought I would sail through college with my athletics and charm. These guys weren't impressed by either.

The others in my keg line were falling out at a fast clip. Most were puking their guts out. "Pete," one of the frat guys said, "you've got to pick up the slack. You're a big boy. You got to take care of that keg."

So, I stepped up to help out my team and proceeded to get trashed. Then they blindfolded us, threw us in a truck, and took us to the cornfields. They made us do all kinds of horrible, ridiculous, crazy, humiliating shit, but I stuck with it like a good pledge.

The next morning, my parents picked me up as promised. At breakfast, Mom asked, "How was last night?"

"Guys, you wouldn't believe it if I told you," I said. "It was hell."

They were both in shock, and Mom was crying as they drove away. I couldn't blame them. It was a surprise to all of us. I guess I didn't think about it too much at the beginning because there was no talk of pledging or hell week or any of that crap. I thought I was already in, but the reality was much different. I felt like a fool, like those guys had been so nice to me at first to get me to join. Then they got a free pass to treat me and the other pledges like trash. There was actually one fellow pledge who was so sleep deprived that he thought he was Jesus Christ. They had to call his parents to come get him and take him out of school for treatment. Bonkers.

I got to play some ball there, but that was a disaster as well. Once, we played a pledge football game against another fraternity. I was still jacked at that point, and we played full tackle WITHOUT PADS. My frat gained a new respect for me because I was an animal on the field. I tore into the other team as the outside linebacker. I'd use the crown of my head and ram the quarterback in the jaw. I was a monster. They'd try to block me, and I'd go around and sprint toward the quarterback again. There was no stopping me.

At one point, the quarterback was bleeding after I sacked him. Then their whole team piled on and I was getting punched and kicked. So, I wiggled my arm loose and started punching back. I made contact with one guy's eye socket and opened it right up. You'd think that would stop the game, but we played on. Then, in the 3rd quarter, after making a tackle, I got nailed in the back of the head, so I swung around and punched the guy behind me. Turned out it was the referee. They had to escort me off the field early so the other team wouldn't jump me after the game. It was intense.

Weeks later, someone called me at the frat house and told me I was getting sued for the referee's medical bills. I went into court without a lawyer and said I thought I was punched in the back of the head. I turned around to defend myself. The judge said if that was my only defense, I had to pay his medical bills. My parents weren't happy about it, but they helped me out and it wasn't cheap. Dad even laughed it off. Onward and upward.

I wasn't sure where the anger was coming from, but everyone knew that they could get a rise out of me because I had such a short fuse. I was not proud of my actions, and I think I knew deep down that I wasn't where I should be. Not only the fraternity, but the school atmosphere just wasn't right for me, and the partying just fueled my frustration.

There was one incident where we were gathered in a room and were forced to eat some of the most disgusting food you can ever imagine. I looked down at it and was nauseated. The other pledges were shoving that mess into their mouths, but I refused. I stood up and said, "No! I'm not touching that, and if anyone has a problem with it, let me know now." A guy came up to my face, ready to confront me. I continued. "I don't give a fuck if you had to do this. I'm not touching that. Period. End of story."

"OK, leave him alone," another guy yelled.

I pushed past them, threw open the door, and heaved a chair over a bunch of trucks in the parking lot. I was so filled with rage because all that treatment from my sister's friends and from my classmates came flooding back and I had reached my breaking point again.

The fraternity president rushed outside. "Pete, settle down. Settle down, man."

"No. This is not me. This will never be me. I'm done. I'm out."

The next week, I moved into a dorm. That first semester in the fraternity house, I probably went to one class. My routine was a recipe for disaster—I'd wake up hungover and my only focus was what we were planning to do that night. I was chasing pretty girls like it was a sport, and because of all the hazing and partying, my health took a nosedive. My athletic, toned, high school physique gave way to a puffy, doughy version of my former self. I think my GPA at the end of the year was .05.

Haig was one of the guys I first met at KU. He was a kindred spirit, and we hit it off as great friends quickly. We bonded over athletics and being individuals. Haig was different, and that is what I loved about him. I was the big, tough football player, and he was the smart, shifty soccer player. Maybe it was frustration we shared, because we both could have probably taken a shot at a pro career but didn't for whatever reason. It was frustrating to feel like we were idle athletes. We wanted to be competitive but found out that could get out of hand quickly. When a good-natured game turns into a brawl, it's not a good sign.

"Haig, this is not for me. I'm not sure why I ended up here, but I've made awesome friends." He knew I was searching for something, for myself, and that Kansas was nothing more than a pit stop on my journey.

To my credit, I didn't totally give up on school. In 1997, I continued to search for a place where I belonged by taking a semester at Front Range Community College in Boulder, Colorado. When I went home to Michigan on a break, a family friend told me about the National Outdoors Leadership School (NOLS), which is a leader in outdoor education. It's a school that teaches mountaineering skills and, more importantly, how to learn about yourself in the process. My friend told me I could get some college credit by going on a month-long wilderness trip. *Where do I sign up?*

After reviewing the programs, I chose a mountaineering session in Alaska, probably because of all the reading I had done about the 49th state. When I got there, it was the exact opposite of the frat house experience. It felt like home immediately. This was more my style, and it was obvious by my attitude. I was at peace and in my element. The stress and anger melted away. I'd traded in team sports and camaraderie for solo adventures, and it fit like a glove.

For the first time, I wasn't such an oddball. Admittedly, I was still an entitled little shit. The first night, we went out into "the field," which is what they called going into the wilderness. We set up our tents and the next morning we got up at 6 a.m. while it was absolutely pissing rain. Everyone was packing up their gear, and I said, "Can't we just wait it out?" That attitude did not go over well, and I quickly realized that I had to pull my own weight and get myself together. And I did.

Experiencing the majestic wilderness of Alaska had me transfixed. I couldn't believe the beauty and raw nature that surrounded me. The majestic mountains and gaping valleys held secrets that I'd never imagined possible. With each step, it was as if the forest was calling me, having a conversation with me, allowing me to see beyond myself. Of course, there was no alcohol, and pot was pretty scarce. About three weeks into our journey, a guy pulled me aside and said, "Pete, I found some pot that I'd forgotten about. You want to partake?"

"Are you kidding me? Sure." And we did, but it was different. It wasn't like before when I felt like I had to have it, or I would lose my mind. This time, it was more of a natural, holistic experience. We were one with the forest and enjoying the benefits of nature's beautiful plant. It gave me a new outlook on almost every aspect of my life. Things just fell into place; and for once, I felt like I belonged.

At one point, our guides put us into small groups and took our tents away. Then, they drew an "X" on a map and said, "We will meet you there in 48 hours. You guys are on your own between now and then. Use the skills we've taught you about how to survive in the wilderness and take care of yourselves."

I was in charge of a group, and at one point we had to cross a river that had dangerous glacial runoff rushing by us. I advised everyone to link arms so that if one person stumbled, the others could pick up the slack. We were about halfway across the river when some of the others wanted to retreat, but I was determined. I stood my ground and said we had to push forward although the pressure of the water was making my trekking poles as weak as noodles. I got everyone to the bank, and then I took the last step and missed my footing. I went face first under the water with my backpack on. My teammates jumped into action and pulled me ashore, but it was a scary reminder of the deceptive dangers hidden behind that Alaskan beauty.

When we met up with the guides, they had a nice fire going. They had put up our tents, added hot rocks from the fire and poured water over the rocks to create a sauna for us. The next thing we knew, all the grime and dirt that we'd accumulated over that month just rolled off us. It was a literal transformation of the changes we all felt inside. We were shedding our old attitudes, our preconceptions, our issues, and our problems. It was one of the most spiritual moments I'd ever experienced.

Then we quickly eased into the freezing cold river to clean our-selves. I'd finally found a place where I felt whole. Where I be-longed. Where I could be myself.

After my NOLS experience, I reflected on what I'd been through—elementary school, the partying teen years, pledging the fraternity—and I had a strong feeling that God had been with me the whole time, even though I hadn't realized it. I did not grow up in a religious house, but I could feel His presence, His gentle way of shepherding me along. I realized that I could have lost my life several times because of my life choices, but I felt like He wanted me to learn from those experiences and live a more authentic, humble life.

When I was around 21, I was living in Telluride because I wanted to be close to the beauty of nature that I'd learned to love. My plan was to regroup and figure out what direction I wanted my life to take. A football buddy from high school had found out that he had a talent for playing the piano, and he'd learned classical music by ear. He graduated from Berke-ley School of Music, and we moved to Telluride together. We were at a bar (that is still there today) and the piano player took a break. My friend asked the owner of the place if he could play for a couple of minutes.

The guy looked at my friend in his punk, skater gear and sneered, "Can you play?"

My friend assured him, "Yes, I can play."

"Let's see what you got."

My buddy jumped on the piano bench and started hitting those keys like the pro he was. The owner was pleasantly sur-prised to say the least. "Which nights would you like to work?"

"I'd love to play for you," he said, "as long as my friend Pete can drink on the house while I'm working."

You can't really ask for a better friend than that. We were living together, and we'd drive into town on the nights he played. As he tickled the ivories, I tossed back top-shelf drinks and had a great time. It was magical. After a couple of months, the owner insisted on modifying the agreement. He still wanted my friend to play, but I could only have one drink on the house, then I was on my own for the rest of the night. He was a smart man.

It was an amazing time and yet another step on my journey to find myself and my place in this world. We were skiing/snowboarding more than a hundred days a year, and I worked at an outdoor shop to make just enough money to get by. We played softball in a league, chased women, and listened to lots of live music. It was all about enjoying life and learning what made us happy. I afforded myself that time to learn and get better and explore all that life had to offer. It was sort of my last blowout before becoming an adult, and I couldn't have asked for a better experience.

Haig would come through whenever he could, and we would connect for some good-natured debauchery. He ended up graduating from Kansas ("just barely" he says), and he liked coming to Telluride so we could follow some of our favorite bands. We went through phases. First, it was the Grateful Dead. We loved going to those concerts because it was an immersive experience. It was pure craziness, and we were both into it.

In 1996, we went on a road trip to the Red Rocks Amphitheater in Morrison, Colorado, to see a Phish show. We camped out with some buddies and even Haig's Siberian Husky for some reason. Being that free and among friends was so liberating, and it felt like the future was ours for the taking. We were all searching for direction and purpose and having fun in the process.

We had an extra ticket for this show, and we traded it for a massive bag of marijuana. "That's the largest amount of pot I've ever seen at one time," Haig said as he tossed the Frisbee. We were extremely popular with the others because we were happy to share our bounty, which is the unspoken creed of those shows. It's a collaborative experience, a single event shared collectively, and that included the party supplies.

Later, Haig and I and whoever else wanted to join decided to jump on the Widespread Panic bandwagon. We were feeling free, and it felt good being with people who understood each other with wordless ease. We'd even connect in other cities whenever a Panic show was announced. "Let's meet up in New Orleans!"

After a while, I decided to go back to Kansas to give college another try. I knew I wanted to get an education; I just wasn't sure where I fit in. I was only there for a couple of weeks when I got a phone call from home. My mom had cancer. The details were a blur, but I was back in Michigan and taking Mom to her chemo sessions, holding her hand, and helping her through radiation. I was doing everything I could to save the one person who had stood by me through all my foolishness. Sometimes, I would have to set my alarm for 3 a.m. to wake her up and make sure she took her pills. I did everything I could to lighten her load. It was a three-year rollercoaster ride of remission and resurgence. Celebration and depression. More celebration and more depression. It was a brutal cycle that seemed to have no end.

At her urging, I returned to my life in Colorado but continued to go back and forth, helping as much as I could. I returned to Telluride for a while and got a call that she had been moved to life support. I was so flustered that whole night, as I was supposed to wake up at 6 a.m. to get on a flight back to Michigan. I woke up late the next morning and missed my flight completely. Luckily, I was able to get on a later flight and I heard that my mom was doing OK in the hospital. Disaster averted!

Her stay in the hospital was a living hell. I would fall asleep there and family members would come in and out, offering any assistance they could. Those were some of the hardest moments of my life because most of the time Mom couldn't talk due to an endotracheal tube shoved down her throat. She'd try to communicate, but I couldn't understand her, which was more frustrating. No matter how much I tried, I couldn't make out the words my mother was trying to communicate. I felt helpless.

"Mom, I can't understand you. Can you write on the chalkboard?" I would hold the board still and it worked at first, but soon her handwriting was shaky, and I couldn't decipher what she was writing. I kept telling her, "I love you, Mom. I'm sorry, I can't understand, but I love you." It killed me. Absolutely killed me.

Our family was gathered around her, and I held her hand as they removed the tube, and she took her last breaths. Those brief moments seemed to last for hours. I couldn't believe I was watching my mother's soul leave her body. During her illness, it was obvious she was sick, but my hope was strong, and I refused to allow myself to imagine anything other than a positive outcome. The minute she took her last gasp of air, my mind went blank. I couldn't process the events taking place before my eyes. I wished I could take her place because I would have done it in a second, but I knew that wasn't God's plan.

Watching her beautiful energy leave her body changed me more than I could have ever imagined. Being in the same room, sharing the same air, and realizing I would be able to continue when she couldn't just gutted me. How could this have happened? Why couldn't I fix it? What did God possibly want me to learn from this?

On November 22, 2000, I lost my best friend. She was the one who'd picked me up when I was down and helped me realize there was more to life than money and status. She encouraged me to be true to myself. She stood up for me in elementary school, cheered for me from the bleachers of the football field, and looked the other way when I was partying out of control. That woman had the ability to let me learn lessons on my own, no matter how much it probably pained her to do so.

Leaving that hospital for the last time, I realized that if I was going to progress through life, I had to regroup and re-establish who the hell I was. I needed to remember what made me happy. I needed to find peace. Like she always told me, I needed to be true to myself no matter what anyone else thought.

I reflected on my time in Alaska and how difficult yet rewarding it was. That's when I decided to move to the last frontier and make a life for myself.

It's what Mom would have wanted.

Chapter Four

Alaska

That life of nonstop partying began to take its toll on my body. I'd always stayed in good shape because of all the sports I'd played. My body and strength were gifts that I'd always taken for granted. I didn't have to work hard for them, so it felt like that's that way I'd always be. I was known as a natural all-around athlete, and I was able to coast on that reputation, but I no longer had a physical outlet for my energy and aggression. Without playing on a team, my body was not being challenged, and it began to show. I'd never wanted sports to define me, but now that they didn't, it made me anxious. Athletic performance had been my identity for so long that I wasn't sure who I was without it. So, even though I was gaining weight and losing muscle, I felt like the same guy on the inside, and I acted like it.

When I was in the fraternity, I'd tried to keep up the image of an athlete. There was one time when a bunch of guys came over and challenged us to play hockey in the gym. It was a modified version without skates, just a bunch of knuckleheads armed with hockey sticks and testosterone. I played fast and aggressive, typical all-star, balls-to-the-wall Pete. It was one of the first times I can clearly remember feeling winded and out of shape. It should have been a wakeup call, but of course, it wasn't. That would have been too introspective for me at the time. I was nowhere near understanding that without putting in the work, my athleticism had a shelf-life that was fast approaching expiration.

When I was first living in Telluride, there was an open tennis tournament held at an exclusive club and, typical of me back then, I decided to sign up. I heard when the head pro and the No. 1 seed were making the draw for matches, the No. 1 seed said, "Who is this Pete Ripmaster? I've never even heard of him. I'll play him in the first round!"

After I heard that, I was even more amped up to compete. I was still in fairly good shape and loaded with well-earned confidence. After not having played in years, there I was taking on the No. 1 seed in the first round of the tournament with a borrowed racket. Looking back, I don't know how I wasn't nervous or hesitant to take this guy on, but I guess that is what brash youth does for you. I barely beat him, but he shook my hand and took the loss like a man.

The day after our match, it was the talk of the town. "Champion takes on outsider with no documented history of wins ... AND LOSES!" Whatever. That just fueled me even more. I even switched up rackets at the last minute because I didn't like the ones most of the players were using. Using a new racket that I had again just borrowed, I performed better than I'd expected. My body didn't let me down, and I went on to win the tournament in a major upset. In the local Telluride newspaper, it said something about a "mystery man" who came from nowhere and defeated the heavy favorites. I'd been in the town for a while, so I didn't consider myself so mysterious, but they had to explain how a novice had trounced the country club star. The attention from that tennis tournament further fueled my confidence.

Around that time, I had to make a roundtrip drive from Denver, Colorado, to Lawrence, Kansas, and back. It was about 560 miles one way, and on the way to Lawrence, I was pulled over by the police. Not shocking.

"You know you're speeding," the stern cop said.

"Sorry, officer."

"Do you have anything in the car that I need to know about?"

"No, sir." I probably did.

"Are you sure?" he persisted.

"I'm sure." I was getting frustrated.

"Why don't you step out of the car."

I got out and he checked my front pockets. There were red, gold, and green rolling papers in my front pocket from when I had been hanging out with my buddies the previous night.

"What are these?" he asked.

I paused and said, "What do they look like?" He didn't find anything else in the car, but I ended up with a fairly significant speeding ticket. That sucked, but I continued to Lawrence. I didn't want to stop before reaching the destination, so I got back on the road to finish the drive. I'd already been traveling for about eight hours at that point, tired but confident that I would soon see the Lawrence exit. I was going through a small town, and it was relatively flat, as was much of the drive, and that lulled me into complacency.

There were no cars in sight, and I had room on both sides of the road so instead of being smart and pulling over, I jumped into the backseat to get something while the car was moving. When I turned back around, the car was veering off the road. I jumped back toward the steering wheel and grabbed it while most of my body was still in the middle row. I severely overcorrected but was able to yank the car away from the sloping shoulder of the road. I pulled over and began to shake. What was wrong with me? What was I thinking? I was pissed at myself, at my cockiness, my reckless behavior, and that feeling of being invincible that stayed with me long after my teenage years.

I was in Telluride in 1999, and I'd been partying as usual, one night after the next. One morning, I was sleeping on a friend's couch after a long night and woke up with a start. I remembered that I needed to get home to take care of my new puppy. I hopped in my car and took off without really thinking about it. I was going fast because I couldn't remember how long it had been since the dog had been out. I looked in the rearview to see blue flashing lights and reluctantly pulled over. The cop instantly smelled last night's regret and gave me a breathalyzer.

"You seem to be fine, but it shows 0.152," he said holding up the digital readout. "Can you say the alphabet backward?"

"Sure," I said. "Just give me a second."

"Never mind," he said. "I'm writing you a ticket. You're obviously still intoxicated." Then he looked me in the eyes. "Listen, this is for your own good. It seems like you've got some major issues that need to be addressed. I suggest you do it."

He wasn't wrong. I actually shook his hand and thanked him as he led me to the backseat of his police vehicle, not for the ticket, but for the concern. He was right about everything.

I was not going to tell my parents about it because I'd been going back and forth while Mom put up a valiant fight against cancer. So, when my court date came up, I went by myself. I had a clean record other than some parking tickets. Despite that, my license was revoked, I spent a couple of days in jail, was required to go to numerous AA classes, and had to perform community service. If I'd been smart, I could have gotten a lawyer to argue for reduced charges, but I was cocky. I was sure that the judge would go easy on me, and that things would work out in my favor, as usual. The fact that she saw through me was certainly a turning point, a slow awakening to the fact that I was not invincible.

And neither was Mom. After losing the most important person in my life, it felt as if my spirit had been crushed. Sorrow washed over me like I'd never experienced before. Everything I did, every thought reminded me of the gaping hole in my life, my new reality. I replayed every conversation, every interaction, trying to maintain a connection, not wanting those memories to fade away. The only relief I found was self-medication.

While I was incredibly close to my mother, there was no denying I had my father's DNA. Seeing how he lived so boldly and unapologetically gave me a sense of empowerment. There was no denying that he was a successful man who lived on his own terms. It worked for him, so I felt like my behavior, no matter how reckless it may have appeared, was justified. "It runs in the family," I'd joke as I built a reputation as a professional partier.

Then after losing Mom, it was like the wheels came off the wagon. That loss gave me more of a reason to indulge, and my friends were even less likely to intervene because of what had happened. It was like I was given a free pass, which now sounds horrible, but in that cloud of pain, it was the perfect emotional storm. A recipe for disaster.

I realized that I needed to make a change. Actually, I needed to make a lot of changes, but I would start with my location. Telluride was my party town, and that was not good for me. After losing Mom, I certainly didn't want to go back home to Michigan. Then, I remembered where I'd felt the most content and serene. I lost my mom in November, and later that winter, I packed up a few belongings and decided to choose my own adventure. That's when I moved to Alaska. By myself.

I could hardly believe that I was finally going to live the dream I'd been thinking about since childhood. Those hours spent reading and rereading books about Alaskan adventures were going to come true. First, I contacted a few people known for dog mushing to see if there was some type of work I could do. That way I could integrate myself into the Iditarod community and fully immerse myself. I also had a Husky I'd raised since he was a pup and brought him along with me. A boy and his dog and the snow.

There was an Iditarod veteran who'd come from Russia, and he was willing to take a chance on me. For some reason, I trusted him right away and was glad for the opportunity. I worked steadily to learn all I could about the dogs, mushing, and everything that goes with it. I was focused and happy to have something that required so much hard work. It felt good, and I loved handling the dogs. Finally, the owner felt like I was ready to run my own dog team. As usual, I was extremely confident in my abilities.

I took out my own team of dogs, only six compared to the typical team of 12 or 16. Still, for me, six was a lot. We took a long loop around the farm and kept going. I found out quickly that it's not easy to manage the sled, and once the dogs were running full bore, I kept leaning left and right, working hard to recover and balance myself.

Somehow, one of the dog harnesses got twisted and two dogs started fighting and nipping at each other. I knew I needed to stop and take care of this before a bigger problem presented itself. I threw the snow hook into the snow to anchor us while I attended to the dogs. As I worked to untangle the harness, I noticed the dogs starting to move. How was that even possible? Then I saw that the hook was not secured, and the sled began to head toward me and the dogs. I knew that if they took off with the sled and without me, they could get wrapped around a tree, hung up in the forest, or worse.

I remembered the No. 1 rule that I'd been taught: Always hang on to your team at all costs. So, I realized right away that I needed to wait and then jump on the sled as it came by me.

Just as it passed, I twisted around and threw my body onto the sled. I didn't realize the snow hook had landed on the back of the sled and it sliced right through my calf, leaving a gaping hole.

I yelled as loud as I could, and I guess the dogs were startled because they stopped immediately. I happened to see the guy who I worked for on a snow machine about three-quarters of a mile away. He saw me frantically waving my arms and came over.

"Pete, you have to take my snow machine and drive it back to the cabin. I'll handle the dogs. I'll get them back to the cabin, but I need to take care of them while you head back."

So, I had to ride a goddamn snow machine back to the cabin as I felt myself going in and out of consciousness. It was the only option, and I knew that this was serious. At the cabin, I elevated my leg, put pressure on it, and I realized that I was not in a good place.

After my boss had put the dogs away, he helped me perform some basic first aid. I was shaking profusely and feeling very alone. *Was this the right thing for me? Had I made a big mistake coming here?* My boss was taking good care of me, but I realized I didn't know anyone else here very well. He called 911 and it took almost two hours for them to arrive. To his credit, he was trying to joke around and keep me distracted, but I was agitated, to say the least.

As I was traveling in the ambulance, one of the attendants pulled my bandage off and gasped. I told them to give it to me straight—what was going to happen? One of the ladies said that amputation was certainly a possibility. That scared the hell out of me. I'd been an athlete all my life, and to have that taken away would be devastating. In the hospital, the doctors said they were going to put me under.

"Not yet," I said. "I want to know what you think first. How does it look?"

Two doctors went to work assessing the damage. "Your leg is torn up, but the tendon was not severed. We should be able to repair this, and then it will need time to heal."

I was ecstatic to be released from the hospital the next day. I took my bandaged leg and a small group of dogs and did a quick lap just to prove to myself that I could do it. When my boss found out, he tried to talk some sense into me, but I was headstrong and determined to prove myself.

"Pete, you are going to be eaten up in this life. I love you to death, but you are too damn naive and far too nice to people. You have to be tough up here or folks will take advantage of you. It's not an easy life."

I realized that he was right. Alaska wasn't where I belonged full-time. I loved being there, but that didn't mean I had to live there, in harsh conditions, carving out a living because there were no other options for me. But it did cause me to reflect on my adventures. It was a crazy time, to be sure. Many nights I'd come home so tired I could barely fire up the single-burner stove. After I had a warm meal, I'd delve into a good book, and everything felt right. I was a regular at the local library and reading about incredible adventures in the middle of my own adventure was a meta experience. How much more adventure did I need?

Maybe I felt some type of affinity for these thrill seekers, like Hudson Stuck, who conquered Mt. McKinley in 1913 and then wrote about it in *The Ascent of Denali*. I enjoyed the renegade life, the cowboy mentality of going it alone. What I started to realize was that even if it wasn't going to be permanent, the Alaskan adventure was exactly what I'd needed. It was humbling and educational. I felt like a tiny speck of dust among the grandeur and expansiveness. It helped to center me and teach me about my limitations as a human being. It was a deep spiritual connection to the wilderness—the explosive colors of the sunrise, the majestic animals that roamed freely.

There were no fancy restaurants, country clubs, or luxury vehicles. It was my school of hard knocks, and it was just what I needed.

I came away from that experience with the beautiful realization that I'll never be defined by the things I own. I was deeper than that, and the Alaskan experience proved it. I also began developing more of a spiritual side. I wasn't completely devoted to Christianity at that point, but the pure beauty of Alaska was clear proof to me that there was much more to life than our existence here on Earth.

That process of stripping away all the distractions helped me process Mom's death and deal with my own demons. My focus was on the tasks at hand, and that helped me prioritize my goals. Drinking and partying all night lost its luster and just seemed like a colossal waste of time after all that I'd experienced in the 49th state.

Before my Alaska adventure, it felt like I was painting my own life of rainbows and sunshine. Everything seemed perfectly arranged, and I didn't want that anymore. I was tired of the pretentiousness and predictability. I'd proved to myself that I didn't need those things to survive, or even to be happy. I had been content in a drafty cabin with a can of beans and a good book. It doesn't get much more stripped down than that. I didn't realize it at the time, but I had learned how to be happy with myself, not with what I had or what was given to me. I learned that putting in the hard work and reaping the rewards, however small, was so much more gratifying, and it gave me joy. It wasn't about finding the right college or being the best athlete or earning the most money. Those things would be a nice bonus for me but not the sole purpose of my life.

Being content and at peace with myself was probably the biggest lesson of all. Loving myself, faults and all, meant I could begin to live an authentic life. I'd always been drawn to people referred to as offbeat or weirdos—poets, artists, writers, gypsies, and musicians. Those were my teachers; their stories are woven into the fabric of my life. Some friends and family members knew where I was in Alaska and emailed occasionally, but it was an eye-opening experience to realize that I was all alone, and no one was there to help me or to fix my mistakes. That isolation forced me to examine some of the things I'd done in the past and decide where I wanted my life to go.

Learning to be self-reliant was invaluable because I'd been so accustomed to comfort. There, I was basically a bum living off the land and loving every minute of it. I loved the challenges, the obstacles, and the toughness because it meant that I was not only capable but that I was my authentic self. And my left calf has a big scar to prove it.

Chapter Five

The Cleansing Snow

Today, when I give talks and presentations about the adventures and challenges in my life, I inevitably get questions from concerned parents about their wayward kids. They are usually talking about a teenager, typically male, who seems to be going down the wrong path or hanging out with a bad crowd. Inevitably, a harried woman or stern-looking man will come up to me and say, "I wish my son were here to listen to you. He's in that teenage phase of being young and selfish. I think hearing you would make such a difference to him."

I always try to reassure those parents, "You have to be patient with your child! Some of them mature later than their peers, and it sounds like yours may be one of those. Just realize that it's OK. A lot of times, I feel those people end up being the most special. Their development is just taking more time than others. My advice is just don't give up. Do the opposite. Give as much love as you can. I understand that might be difficult because teenagers can be annoying as hell, but I was in the same spot. I think my mother's constant effort to get through to me eventually saved me from myself."

It's true. I was just like those kids, feeling like I didn't belong anywhere. My family and friends loved me, but I felt an emptiness and a disconnect that I didn't completely understand. I was never a "bad" person and never out to hurt anybody. I was just searching—always searching. I wanted something deeper and more meaningful, but what did that mean? I wasn't sure but had a deep-seated feeling that I would find out in my lifetime.

There was no denying that while I could assimilate with my peers when I wanted to, I was basically a misfit, a loner, an outlier. Most of my friends went on to college for four years, got their first professional job after graduation, and began pairing up and starting families. It was happening all around me at an alarming pace. It felt as if they were passing me by, and that only helped to feed my feelings of isolation. At that age, their focus was on that important first job and building a career, often one that required many hours of dedication, something young workers are usually eager to provide.

Then there was me, around 24 or so, with no college degree, no clear career direction, no mother, and no serious relationship. My life was stuck in neutral as everyone else was laying on the gas pedal, zooming down their own career path with palpable excitement and zeal. Naturally, their free time and inclination to party were drastically curtailed by the demands of their careers. The growing chasm between me and everyone else was impossible to ignore, and it only fed into those dark feelings of seclusion and detachment that bubbled up with increasing frequency.

I felt like the protagonist of a sad story, a cautionary tale of a young man who had so much promise and all the socioeconomic advantages anyone could want and had pissed it all away. With my mother gone, I was just floating through life. I wanted to have the career drive my friends had, and I wanted to be excited to go to an office every day and grow my career. I wanted all those things, but I just couldn't do it. There were times when I'd think about the good times in high school, the cheers from the crowd when I scored a touchdown, that feeling of endless possibilities. I started to realize if I was reminiscing about the good times when I was only in my early twenties, there was a definite problem. It was clear that my path would not be a typical one.

After my mother passed away, our family center was gone and the rest of us were left to fend for ourselves. We had a huge church service for her, and after that it was clear that our family would never be the same. However, we did try to stay connected in our own way. Dad was definitely at a loss even though he wouldn't admit it. My sister had the idea that the four of us needed to go on a trip. The first suggestion was Turks and Caicos. Not only was I still broken up from losing Mom, but a tropical island held no appeal for me. I was never a beach person, so I couldn't imagine anything worse than sitting in the hot sand and missing my mother. No, thank you.

"The mountains are what brings me peace," I told them. "I need to go back to Telluride. I have some friends there, not to mention my dogs."

They understood, but there was no denying that Dad's mood was going downhill without Mom around. He was clearly not handling it well. As the oldest son, the family looked to me for guidance. I wanted to be strong for them, but the truth was that I just couldn't. I had already been trying to figure out my direction in life and now my mother was gone. I'd been there when she took her last breath, and then it was over. How could a life be extinguished so suddenly? How could an entire family be turned upside-down in a split second?

I felt guilty leaving them to their own devices, but they understood and decided to move forward with their plans to vacation together as a way to handle the aching loss we all felt. My friends were excited about my return, and so was I. When I got back to Telluride, it was refreshing to be greeted with such warmth after going through such loss. These were my pals, and they were excited to see me and eager to help me cope with my new reality.

"How can we help you?" one of them asked. "What can we do?"

"To be honest," I said, "I could really use a hike in the mountains by myself. I just need some peace and quiet."

They were understandably concerned. "Are you sure that is what you want? We're here for you, man. We will help you through this."

"If you want to help, just let me do this. Let me take my dogs and hike for a little while. I promise it will be OK. I'll just be gone for a few hours."

They all agreed that I had to handle things in my own way, and I appreciated their concern. It also felt good to be back in a more relaxed atmosphere. Telluride is a tourist town, so the locals weren't saddled with unchecked career drive. Their focus was on enjoying the moment and emphasizing friendship over job promotions. That's just what I needed.

It was a sunny, brisk December day, the kind of day where the sky is so blue it almost hurts to look at. No matter how hard I tried, I couldn't locate a single cloud. A thin layer of snow covered the ground, adding to the serene feeling of the majestic mountain. In a matter of minutes, I was hiking up Bear Creek with my northern-breed dogs wagging their tails and trotting along beside me. I couldn't have been more in my element. With each crunch of snow, I could feel the healing powers of nature wash over me. It was nothing short of magical.

At one point, I reached a clearing and decided to take a minute to soak it all in. There wasn't a soul around. I think most were up on the slopes with the tourists. That was fine with me because it gave me time to acclimate to my surroundings, my adopted home. I could hear the gurgling of the small creek that ran parallel to the trail. My excited pups became distracted by a critter and ran off toward the water.

The forest became completely still. The wind stopped blowing. Leaves settled on their branches. The sounds of the birds faded into the ether. I couldn't even hear the melodic water bouncing along the rock-filled stream. Sheer quiet. I looked up at the sky, still smooth and clear. I realized that the only movement, the only thing that was not still, not at peace, not comfortable in its own being, was me. Then without warning, a single tear trickled down my cheek.

The waterworks came without notice, and I started crying uncontrollably. I felt claustrophobic in my own skin, and I took a seat on the downed tree beside me on the trail. Tears were flowing down my face so fast that I couldn't see, couldn't get my bearings. I heard a strange, shrill scream and realized it was coming from me. I looked up at the pine trees swirling around me. I tried to find a focal point that I could concentrate on to try and control my breathing, but it was no use. The forest was a flurry of greens and browns surrounding and sheltering me as I sat.

I thought, *Calm down, Pete. You just need to breathe. Focus on your breathing.* Just then, I looked off to the side and there was a beautiful tree that captivated me for some reason. I looked at it from afar and sort of tilted my head from side to side, like an inquisitive dog. I studied the tree and felt a very real connection to it. I focused on controlling my breathing, and I started to relax. I could feel the weight on my shoulders ease, and I noticed the birds were singing once again. I scanned the forest for a sign of my dogs, but they were nowhere to be found. Next, I again returned my attention to this huge, mystical pine tree coated in snow only about 30 yards away.

For some reason, I felt a strong connection to the sturdy tree on that snowy mountain. Maybe it was the shape of the trunk or the way the branches were arranged. I was inexplicably drawn to the tree. I couldn't take my eyes off it. It seemed fully alive and extremely powerful.

Out of nowhere, a gust of wind rushed from behind the tree and blew a burst of snow in my direction. As I sat there, the gentle, glistening snow fell all around me, covering my head, my shoulders, and finally, my face. I closed my eyes and felt the frosty flakes land on my warm skin and drip down my neck. It felt like a cleansing, a renewal, a rebirth. I had been washed.

I didn't shield my face or turn away in the slightest. I stayed open to the experience and remained still, allowing it to happen organically. I stretched my hands upward, welcoming it, embracing the moment. I remember closing my eyes and feeling as if the snow was actually going through me, like it was pelting my face and then boring its way inside, cooling me before it left as quickly as it had arrived. It was an energy, a spirit, a consciousness like I'd never felt before. It was as if I had been chosen, singled out for the experience.

Once I processed what had happened, it made me smile, and then I broke out into a laugh. I felt the pure joy that had consumed me and washed away the pain I'd brought with me up the mountain. It was as if a presence was there, one that felt familiar. One that felt like my mother.

As quickly as it came, the flurry of snow was gone, and the air cleared. I stood up and felt a lightness and happiness that I'd never felt before. My face ached so I reached up to feel it and realized that I was smiling and had been for a while. My happy dogs appeared out of the brush and stood panting by my side. I patted their warm fur and started back down the mountain as their tails whacked my legs with each step.

When I got to the bottom, my friends were glad to see me and asked how the hike was. I didn't know what to say. How could I explain something like that? "It was amazing," I said.

It wasn't too long after that when I got down on my knees in my basement and said, "Jesus, I am yours. This life is too hard for me on my own." What I thought to be my mother's spirit was actually a Holy Spirit moment. What I realized at that moment was that He had been with me my whole life, I just hadn't truly realized it. I had the Holy Spirit looking after me even though I wasn't sure that I deserved it. I was slowly learning that's the real beauty of faith. It's there for you; it's not something that you work toward. It is given freely. Once I realized that, it changed my life forever and continues to be a foundational part of who I am.

Even today, years later, with a family of my own, I continue to have my issues with depression, making choices I regret or saying something I wish I hadn't, but I've learned to be patient with myself. I am a work in progress. I think we all are. I'll never be that perfect person I imagine in my head, but that's OK. Now, I understand that I can make mistakes and live a bold life because I have faith and trust in God.

As part of my spiritual journey, I started going to churches, but many of them didn't feel right to me; they didn't inspire me the way I needed. I had several friends offer up their churches for me to try, and I was eager to do it. I was searching for the best place for me and my family to worship, so I had to do my research. However, time and again, all the beautiful churches with lovely services still weren't right. I was determined to trust my instincts. I knew that I would know when the right fit came along.

During my morning runs in my adopted town of Asheville, North Carolina, I used to pass a missionary Baptist church that was predominantly African American. One day as I passed, I heard the most beautiful music wafting from its interior. It had such a strong pull on my soul that I stopped running and slowly walked to the door. The music was louder and more mesmerizing the closer I got, so I opened the door and went inside.

The bright sunlight drenched the congregation, and they all turned to see my silhouette with my hands outstretched, holding open the doors wide. It was a humble one-room building filled with worshippers dressed in their finest, the pews dotted with men in dapper suits and ladies wearing beautiful, ornate hats. I slipped into a pew at the back and the churchgoers gradually returned their attention to the pastor stationed behind the podium. I'd totally forgotten that I was in my workout clothes, fresh from a sweaty run, so I must have looked like a hound dog that had been playing in a creek.

I needn't have worried about my appearance though, because after the service so many people came up to introduce themselves. They welcomed me to their hallowed church with open arms. Ladies gushed over me, and men shook my hand heartily. They hugged me and loved on me like I was an old friend. I'd never felt such acceptance and pure openness as I did at that moment. I could feel the presence of Jesus. I could feel the spirit and the truth of it all, and I realized at that moment how much I'd been missing before I accepted Jesus.

I returned several times in the weeks that followed, even bringing my daughter to experience the singing and dancing and fellowship. I also took vegetables and other bounty to share with anyone who wanted to partake. Later, my family found a church closer to our home that worked for us, but I'm not sure if I would have ever found the right place if I hadn't experienced the beauty and love of that small rural church that opened my soul and reaffirmed my faith. They welcomed me without judgment about my past or the fact that I looked different than most of them. It was an important part of my spiritual growth.

Today, I've settled into my faith. I'm still kind of a loner. My church is a place where I feel comfortable attending when

I am home, but even more importantly, I don't beat myself up when I can't go because of my running/speaking schedule. I've learned that there is no one-size-fits-all religion and that it doesn't have to look a certain way. How I choose to worship works for me, and I've come to realize that I don't have to put on a facade or pretend I'm something that I'm not. I can be myself and have Jesus in my life.

Granted, I got a late start in my spiritual journey, but that's what worked for me. Since I've embraced my faith, I feel like I've made better decisions and my life has evolved into something that I'm proud of, that I truly enjoy. Even when the darkness creeps in—which it often does—I remind myself that there is light and hope and beauty in life. There will always be sad times, but the difference is that now I understand that's only temporary. I'll come out on the other side wiser and better than before.

One of the biggest lessons I learned is that I cannot worry about what other people think about me. My focus needs to remain on my family and my direct relationship with God, Jesus, and the Holy Spirit. While I'm far from perfect and have made some mistakes I surely needed to repent for, I feel like I'm on the right path, that I'm working toward being the best person I can be. To me, that means not only being good to myself but treating others with kindness and respect. When I instinctively rejected the crowd mentality of bullying as a teen or refused to go along with behavior that I felt was wrong, that was a core part of my spiritual makeup that I didn't realize at the time. I'd made plenty of poor decisions and bad choices, but when it came down to it, I always had the strength to stay true to my core beliefs.

Developing the spiritual part of my life helped me put things into context and make sense of some of the decisions I'd made. It also gave me the confidence to say that I am a good person just the way I am. If someone doesn't like me or wants to change me, I can acknowledge that, but I need to stay true to myself. I am certainly not your "typical Christian." I sometimes cuss like a sailor. Lord knows I've drunk one too many beers and flirted with too many pretty girls. And I often quote this Waylon Jennings lyric: "If my good's a pound, my bad must be a ton."

There's no denying that I've had things handed to me, and I've been so blessed in so many ways; but to be honest, I was just as happy in a snow-covered shack in Alaska as I was in a McMansion in the suburbs. I used to beat myself up about that. I'd feel guilty that my family was well-off when so many others struggled. When my faith came into focus, things began to make sense. I realized that I couldn't change my circumstances, but I could make thoughtful choices about helping others. I learned that if I'm authentic to myself and to my faith, my life is much more fulfilling and richer.

My spiritual journey truly began on that rocky mountain path in Telluride when the Holy Spirit washed over me. This awakened in me the belief that there is something beyond myself and my problems. This experience opened my heart and my mind to infinite possibilities about the wonders that lay ahead for me, including meeting the love of my life. I'm not sure if I would have been open to that if I hadn't had that moment high in the San Juan Mountains. Life was sure becoming colorful.

Chapter Six

To Hell You Ride

Telluride was the sweet spot for me. It wasn't as remote and isolating as Alaska, and not as emotionally smothering as Michigan. The town was permeated with a sense of anticipation and adventure, and that's what I needed after experiencing such a loss in my life. Thrill seekers came from all over to test their mettle on the formidable slopes and challenging trails. Others were content to soak in the atmosphere, enjoy the majestic scenery, and leave their everyday lives far behind. Cathedral mountains welcomed everyone to enjoy nature's gifts. Those simple joys had the power to transform a person with breathtaking scenic views or a glimpse of a hawk soaring through the chilly morning air.

The joyful exuberance of the town juxtaposed with the quiet solitude of the winding trails had me wrapped up in a protective cocoon of comfort. I was equally happy shooting the shit at a local bar or talking to God as I watched silver clouds dance across the western sky. The pureness of the mountains had a healing effect on me. It was a time for me to readjust my thinking and press reset on my life. I wasn't sure where my life was headed, and without my mom around, I felt more alone than ever.

Career-wise, I was about as focused as a squirrel in the middle of a busy road. I had an assortment of jobs that kept me busy and made a little money. I worked at an outdoor shop for a while, and then I took a job as a camp counselor. I entered each new position thinking it would be the perfect fit for me and that I was going to make a real difference. I went into the outdoor camp with lofty ideas of sharing my outdoor knowledge with kids who would be held in rapt reverence as I dispensed valuable knowledge about how to purify water or stay warm in a snowstorm. Sometimes, the job fulfilled me; other times I felt like a glorified babysitter. The change of seasons was one of the only things to keep me inspired, though, as Telluride afforded a plethora of outdoor opportunities. On any given day, you could find me mountaineering, fishing, rock climbing, ice climbing, playing softball, Frisbee, golf, tennis, skiing, or enjoying a cold beer (or six) at a favorite local watering hole!

Social life in the small town was an interesting mix of easygoing locals amid a constant stream of carefree visitors looking for temporary thrills before returning to their jobs and bills and responsibilities. I ran into locals at all the bars I walked into, and of course, we could spot the out-of-towners right away. My posse regularly set its sights on beautiful ladies who were looking for a little fun at 8,750 feet in elevation.

In 2003, the MTV show *Real World/Road Rules Challenge: The Gauntlet* was filming in Telluride (also known as "To Hell You Ride"). I didn't watch a lot of TV, but I'd seen enough of MTV to understand what the show was about. Of course, it was the talk of the town because a film crew was taking over various areas to shoot elaborate contests and drinking games. It was a good location for that type of show because of the outdoor amenities and the party atmosphere of the town. The cast from the show was a combination of testosterone-filled guys and ambitious girls trying to compete in challenges while looking good for the camera. Naturally, they infiltrated the bars and restaurants around town with camera guys and boom mics in tow.

I was working at yet another job; this time it was a liquor store. It wasn't at all challenging, but it was the one place almost everyone in town came to visit. So, I was able to fraternize with my buddies and keep tabs on the newbies. The MTV guys came in occasionally and seemed like glorified frat boys, but I didn't know if they were really that clueless or if they were playing to the cameras. Either way, it was good for a laugh and gave us something to talk about.

From the liquor store, I had a bird's eye view of Main Street, and at one point, I saw a tall, beautiful woman I'd noticed around town walking with one of the *Road Rules* guys. I'd heard that she had relocated from North Carolina recently, but I hadn't been able to talk to her. I told my buddies that I hoped she would come into the store or that I'd get the chance to talk to her at a bar. Now, seeing her with Mr. MTV, I figured my chances were over. Maybe she was impressed because he was on TV. If that was the case, I was better off knowing that.

The next morning, I stumbled into a restaurant to sober up from the night before. I needed coffee and some breakfast before my shift at the store began. I was squinting to focus on the words of the menu when I heard a voice beside me.

"Hey y'all, Good morning. Can I get you something?"

I looked up, and it was the girl I'd seen the day before. I hadn't realized she was working there. "Hey, it's you. How's it going?" I said, trying not to sound too enthusiastic.

"I'm good. Can I get you something to drink?"

"Sure," I said with a smile. "I think I'll have a whiskey and water."

"You do know it's 8:45 in the morning, right?"

"Yeah, I know. Will you just see what you can do, please?"

I was testing my luck. She probably thought I was an alcoholic or something, but I was curious to see how she would react.

Soon she was back at the table. "The bar isn't open right now, but I got someone to fix a drink for you anyway."

That was all she had to say. I was sprung, hooked, smitten, whatever you want to call it. I wish I could truly describe the feeling of instant chemistry that we had. There were so many unknowns in my life, so many things went unanswered; but for once, I was completely sure about how I felt. I loved her confidence, and it was obvious that she wouldn't put up with a lot of bullshit. I was a sucker for someone who seemed authentic and self-assured.

When I'd seen her around town with her cute friend, they were always surrounded by guys eager to ply them with whiskey and compliments. That was never my style, so I always hung back, watched the interaction, and wished I were aggressive enough to push my way through the crowd and turn on the charm. That just wasn't me. I was never good at letting people know how I felt about them. It may have been out of fear that I'd get too close and lose them. Maybe it went back to being ostracized as a kid. I'm not sure, but I just wasn't the guy who was going to fight over a girl. Never gonna happen.

The dating pool was stacked against me from the beginning because there were many more guys in town than girls. I guess the single women paired up pretty quickly and settled down or moved out of town. So, if I were interested in someone, there would definitely be competition, and that meant I'd retreat and let the chips fall where they may. There were several times when I watched guys go up to this girl and her friend, eager to buy them drinks all night long. I'd sit back and watch the spectacle, mentally checking her off the list of potential dates.

Naturally, everyone talks in a small town, and I'd found out that her name was Kristen, and her friend was Audrey. The two of them had recently moved to Telluride because Kristen's older brother, John, had been spending time there. Kristen had recently graduated from UNC-Greensboro, and the word was that she wanted to have a little singleton fun with her friend before being strapped into a full-time job on the first rung of the corporate ladder.

I couldn't believe that I was having a liquid breakfast served by this tall, southern beauty who I'd seen in the bars, not to mention in the company of a "reality star." Finally, she was focused on me and there were no other dudes jockeying for her attention. I left that restaurant with the satisfaction that Kristen knew who I was and that we definitely had some type of connection, at least on my part.

I stayed busy chasing adventure, chasing a buzz, and chasing music. In fact, the music scene was surprisingly active for a small town, especially during tourist season. I had a friend who worked at KOTO, the local radio station, so I was always the first to know about new music and upcoming tours. When I found out Widespread Panic was coming to town, I was beyond psyched. Their music had gotten me through some painful times in my life, and I often listened to them as I hiked the woods. I was stoked when my buddy at the station said he'd try to arrange for me to meet the band. They were playing for two nights, and I was like a little kid at Christmas. I couldn't wait to see them jam, live in my small mountain town. So cool.

My friend said, "I have a way that you can meet the band."

"Ok great," I said. "How's this going to work?"

"I set it up, so you'll be the person to take care of their contract rider."

"Rider? What does that mean? I just want to meet them."

I didn't realize I'd have to work at the concert! I just wanted to say hey to the guys. My friend handed me several pages of paper that detailed everything the band requested while they were in town. It was A LOT.

This was a time when I was barely able to take care of myself. How the hell was I supposed to look after a group of rock stars? A couple of days before the concert, as reality set in, I told them, "I'm out completely. I'm just going to go to the show like everybody else, and I'm not going to worry about backstage. Forget trying to meet the band. I'm just gonna enjoy the music like everyone else."

Following my instincts was the way to go because on the night of the show, I was having a great time—shirt off, arms up, buzz on, just dancing to the music. Suddenly, I looked to my left, and there was the waitress from the restaurant, Kristen. I couldn't believe my luck. There were no guys surrounding her like she usually had. It was a sign.

We talked and danced from one song to the next, just enjoying the chill vibe and getting to know each other. I could feel the attraction immediately. The chemistry was undeniable. Then I turned to my left for just a minute and when I looked back, she was leaving the concert with another guy. What the hell? Where did he come from? I couldn't believe it because it was obvious there was a connection between us. We even talked about hanging out after the show was over and now this?

I ran into her in town the next day and confronted her. I was still shocked that she'd bailed after we'd had such a good time. And to leave with another dude, that was just too much, so I wanted some answers.

"I thought we were having a good time at the show," I said. "What's up? You left with another guy. How could you do that?"

"You mean my brother?"

At that moment, I could feel the anger leave my body. I was ready to tell her how inconsiderate she had been and then found out that she'd gone to the concert with her brother, and he needed to leave. She'd planned to tell me about it later, but

I hadn't given her the chance. That's because I'd decided to be uncharacteristically aggressive and tell her how I felt.

"You know, I'm leaving town soon. I'm heading to Missoula, Montana. I had a great time with you last night, and I'd like to take you out." I held my breath and waited for a response.

She smiled. "I'd like that."

I couldn't believe my luck. I realized that I needed to get my life together if I was going to try and make this work. At that moment, I was nearly living paycheck to paycheck. A few nights after that, we were all at the bar and I wanted to impress Kristen and her friends.

"I'm going to pay for everyone's drinks!" I announced.

"Are you sure?" Kristen asked.

"Of course."

"OK, thank you. We'll pay the tip."

"Nope. I'll take care of that, too!" Man, I was feeling generous. There's no easier way to make friends at a bar, and I wanted her friends to like me. The only problem was that I had about $100 to my name. I snapped my card down in front of the bartender.

"Uh, this card was declined."

Dammit! "Here, try this one," I said as confidently as possible.

"This one doesn't work either."

By combining what I had in my pocket with a little from each card, I was able to pay the tab. Fortunately, I was on the other side of the bar and the ladies were none the wiser.

"OK, folks. The tab is paid. No problem at all!"

It was to be a humble beginning for us, but that was fine as far as I was concerned. I have always gone on intuition and the assumption that everything will work out somehow. She didn't know anything about where I came from, and I didn't know much about her life. We were starting with a clean slate. Neither of us had expectations beyond what was right in front of us. With love and patience, our lives would come together, and we'd begin this journey in life, side by side. She clearly understood that I was a free-spirited, good-natured guy looking for my next adventure, and she was a beautiful, fun, educated woman ready to start a career.

I was proud of myself because I'd set out to meet Kristen and followed through with it. Before, if things got too difficult, I would just bail because I knew something else would come along; but this was different. She was different. She was worth pursuing. It was one of the first times that I wasn't prepared to give up without giving it my best shot. *Peter, don't be fucking stupid. Do not mess this up!*

There was never an assumption on my part that it would be easy, or that it wouldn't take work, but that was fine by me. I'd finally found someone who meant something to me. Kristen was the first person I could imagine being with for the long haul. I'd had my share of fun and wild times. While I knew there were still plenty of adventures to be had, I also knew that I wanted to have them with her.

Chapter Seven

All In

Having the feeling that my life was coming together gave me a renewed confidence that I didn't need to follow the traditional paths that my friends and classmates had followed. I'd often go on long runs with friends like Haig, and we'd discuss how our lives were evolving.

"You've definitely changed," he said. "Finding someone seems to have channeled that aggression and competitiveness. You had a bit of a hole after losing your mom. You're coming out of that pain cave and into the light."

That guy has seen me through the crazy fraternity years, the concert phase, and now, a time when I'd finally made a choice about who I wanted to be with for the long haul. It was interesting to see how our lives were growing and evolving.

With my life changing, I was seeking less immersive thrills. I wasn't sure going on trips and long runs were good for my new relationship. Then along came online gambling. It was the wild west of the Internet, and entrepreneurial geeks were trying to find ways to monetize this new, digital world. The online "casinos" that were created pale in comparison to the sophisticated software today. Back then, games consisted of progressive jackpots, themed slot machines, and "tables" where multiple players could have a virtual seat to play a few hands of blackjack.

Following the casinos, online sports betting was gaining popularity. Those sites ran promotions and cash-back offers to entice betters to this new way of placing a wager in hopes of winning big. Then came peer-to-peer betting where people could bet between each other, and even live betting that followed a sporting event in real time.

By that time, I realized that I had an addictive personality, but I don't think I'd come to terms with it. Being addicted to the outdoors or adrenaline sports was different because it was considered a positive way to spend time. Being addicted to a substance or a destructive behavior, however, was another matter entirely.

I'd dabbled in the online gambling world a little bit before I met Kristen, and before I knew it, all I could think about was my next bet. It was not something I completely hid, but I was discreet about it.

With gambling, I started off slowly. It was pure fun. It made me feel connected to sports, something I'd missed, and maybe I still regretted not pursuing an athletic career when I had a chance. Gambling seemed to fill that void. Those first few wins were amazing experiences. They gave me a shot of adrenaline that made me feel alive. I felt part of something big, and it was an exciting outlet at a time when I was trying to figure out what life as a couple would be like. Kristen didn't mind at first. It wasn't something we did together, but she was happy when I won, and more importantly, she was glad I was doing something I enjoyed. And I didn't have to train for weeks and leave home to do it. I would even occasionally buy her something extravagant just because.

"Where'd this come from?" she'd ask.

"I just wanted to get you something special."

Like all addictions, gambling can only be hidden for a limited amount of time. No matter how skilled someone is or how good they cover up something they are not proud of, it has a way of rising to the surface, and that's what my gambling did in our relationship. The destructive finger of addiction wagged in our faces, daring us to slap it away.

Kristen is rather intuitive, and she quickly saw the warning signs. It got to the point where I was intercepting the mail like a crazed postal worker so I could stash credit card statements and hide promotional mailings from companies eager to take the money I didn't have to lose. With my mother gone, there was less control over my investment account, and that access made me somewhat of a high roller. My dad was happy to cosign when needed because his philosophy had always been to live life without railings, no holds barred, guns a-blazing.

I was an immature young man without checks and balances. The problem wasn't that I could not pay my quickly mounting debts; it was that I was getting sucked in, deeper and deeper. No matter how much I won or lost, it was never enough. I needed more. I had to recapture that winning feeling and avoid the despair I felt when I lost. It was an online rollercoaster ride that wouldn't end.

Soon, I was receiving letters touting discounts and even free trips if I would keep adding money to my online account. It wasn't long before I was known as a full-fledged gambler. That was fine, at first. I talked about it openly and shared my excitement when I won. As I got more involved, I stopped talking about it and even began to hide it—not just from Kristen, but friends and family as well. I was embarrassed by how easily I'd been sucked into a world that I knew was only going to become darker and darker.

Lying became an automatic response to any questions about the "hobby" I'd initially been excited about. If anyone asked, I'd assure them that I wasn't really into it anymore.

That was especially true of Kristen. I was so embarrassed that I couldn't quit, so I convinced her that I had given it up, just like that.

Without her knowledge, I was putting large bets on the line, amounts I knew would cause alarm if she had any idea about them. We were a young couple struggling to get established, so disposable income didn't exist. Yet here I was, sneaking onto the computer to place my bets before cutoff time.

It began as all addictions do: gradually. I'd put $500 in an account and bet maybe $50 on a game. That was fun for a short time, but then I needed more. It got to the point where I didn't feel the rush of adrenaline unless there was $1,000 or more on the line. I knew it was risky, and that was the thrill. I was sure that I could beat the system. Sometimes I'd win and it was amazing, but the depression that accompanied a loss became increasingly painful. The only relief was to bet more. There were days when I'd gamble $5,000 or $10,000.

I had an established relationship with one of the larger on-line casinos that offered deals and promotions to keep me gambling. They would make it as tempting as possible. So, I would deposit more money in response and enjoy the perks they lavished on me. One day, they called the house phone.

"Hello?"

"Peter, we have a great deal for you! Because you are one of our favorite customers, we're giving you an all-expenses-paid first-class trip to the Bahamas. We pay for everything: flight, hotel, food, drinks, everything. Bring your wife and have a great time, on us."

"The Bahamas?" I said.

"You will love it. We are inviting a group of our high rollers for this exclusive trip. It will be amazing. We will have new games that our guests can bet on. It's only for a select group. What do you say?"

"Listen. I don't think I can be clearer. I don't want a trip, especially not with my wife. She's not too—well, she doesn't know I'm still using my account. I sure as hell can't go to a tropical island with other gamblers and leave her in a room while I bet on even more games than I already do!"

"I'm not sure you understand. This is all expenses paid. You have nothing to lose."

"Listen. I don't need your 10% discount, and I don't need your free trips. I'm good with the online betting and it ends there. OK?"

It soon got to a point where the winning and losing really had no bearing on my mood. If I lost a little bit or won a small amount, the feeling was more or less the same. I got off on the action. That's what I was after. *Oh my gosh, it's come down to the last second. If he misses this free throw, I'm going to lose it!*

There were times when I'd win six, seven, or eight games in a row. I'd be on a winning streak and win maybe $15,000. I'd think of all the things I could buy, or the good things I could do with that money if I cashed in. I'd entertain all the scenarios but would ultimately return to the same action: Let it ride.

Then I'd make promises to myself that I knew I wouldn't keep. *I'll just do one more game. This time, if I lose, I'll definitely stop.* When I did start losing, I'd watch the account dwindle down to just a few thousand dollars, and that feeling of depression would take hold. I'd feel embarrassed and guilty because I knew I should have stopped when I was ahead. It seemed so logical, but I couldn't follow through with my plan.

That cycle of winning and losing, especially when it was online, had a way of taking away the actual value of money. I started to lose touch with what that amount of money meant. I would rationalize everything as long as it meant I could keep betting.

One time, I was down to about $3,000 in my account. It somehow became crystal clear how much money I'd lost over the past several weeks. That was it for me... almost. I decided, *I'm just going to pick the biggest underdog of the whole freaking sportsbook tonight. And I'm going to put $3,000.00 on the biggest underdog, and I'm just going to let it ride. Then I'll be at zero, and I can stop. I don't care anymore. This is just too much.* Rationally, I could have just stopped and withdrawn the balance from my account, but an addict doesn't think quite so clearly.

I bet $3,000 dollars on a Nebraska basketball team that was absolutely terrible. The Cornhuskers were given 22 points and I actually chose Nebraska to WIN the game, not just cover the massive point spread. It was a huge spread, so statistically, it was a ridiculous bet where I was basically giving my money away. That was fine with me because I was truly at the end of my rope. I wanted it to stop, but I needed it to happen with a big loss. Somehow, I had justified to myself that it was better that way.

Kristen knew nothing of my antics. I'd assured her that it was all behind me, and I'd hidden any postal evidence to the contrary. It felt like I was home free. One last stupid game and I'd be finished with this secret part of my life. I could stop the guilt and secrets that were bottled up inside me.

We were in bed around 11 p.m. that night and I was just about to fall asleep when the sports announcer came on. I couldn't focus on what he was saying because I was reading the ticker crawling along the bottom of the screen. It was the game I'd bet on, and Nebraska was down by only one point. What the hell?

I could feel my pulse begin to race, and I was certain my heart was pounding loud enough to be heard. I stole a quick look at Kristen, but she was busy with a magazine, paying absolutely no attention to the TV.

The next thing I knew, I saw that Nebraska had WON on a last second shot. I stared at the TV in disbelief. I'd won more than $20,000, and I was suddenly, once again, filled with that rush of adrenaline. This time, I couldn't show it. I stayed as still as possible. Then I went to the bathroom and screamed into a towel. I was buoyed by the excitement but had no outlet.

That should have been a time of celebration, but I couldn't do that because it was a secret. I realized that it wasn't worth it. I was at the point where even if I did win, I couldn't express it, and I certainly couldn't spend the winnings. The only alternative would be to bet it all again and continue the cycle, and I just couldn't go through with that anymore.

I crawled back into bed and looked at Kristen, who was still reading her magazine. It was going to be the end of the secrets. I'd no longer have to live a life shrouded in secrecy. To be honest, the whole thing had become exhausting. It took a lot of energy to hide that part of my life, and I was relieved to let it go. I eventually told Kristen everything and happily assured her that it was behind me.

After closing all my accounts, I was proud that I'd conquered that online demon once and for all. With my personality, I knew I'd have to find other ways to enjoy life as a couple, and I was sure that was possible. Kristen and I were ready to begin our careers and carve out a life on the east coast. Professional jobs would leave little time for much else, so I was ready to get started.

Chapter Eight

Teaching the Teacher

Aside from the shock and sadness that inevitably comes from losing someone you love, death can sometimes also give new life and spur major inspiration in those left behind. I didn't realize it at the time, but that's what happened to me after my Grandpa Dobson passed away in 2003. He was an integral part of my life and a source of advice and wisdom. Once it hit me that he was gone for good, I looked at my life and made some decisions. I had already lost my grandma and grandpa Ripmaster who had had brought so much love, laughter, and color to my life. Mom was gone too. Regardless, things were now moving in the right direction. It was high time for me to pick up the pieces and spread my wings. I'd met Kristen and knew already that she was going to be an important part of my life. I also realized that I needed to focus on a career. Working with kids in Telluride gave me a sense of satisfaction, and that was going to be my focus. I'd long ago prepared my family for the fact that I had no interest in pursuing a corporate life, so I think Grandma Dobson, Kristen, and everyone else was happy with my decision to become a teacher.

Kristen was settling into a career in sales after landing a job in Asheville, North Carolina. First, I enrolled at the University of North Carolina-Asheville (UNCA), but it didn't seem like the right fit. Since I'd been bouncing around colleges and taking time off to work, I was older than most students in my classes. Normally, that would have been fine with me because I was used to being an outlier, but I was no longer interested in talking to my classmates about keg parties and hangovers. Kristen had a friend who was a guidance counselor, and she had a suggestion for me.

"Pete," Kristen said, "I talked to my friend and told her that you want to be a teacher, but that UNCA wasn't the right fit for you. She said to look into Montreat College."

"Where is that? I've never heard of it," I replied. "But I'll check into it."

One thing that I realized early on, especially for me, was that life's journey is not linear. We have ideas in our head about the path we should follow, maybe because of our parents or someone else who is important in our lives. Then we map it out and maybe even establish arbitrary milestones we hope to achieve—college after high school, graduation in four years, more school or an entry-level job to begin a career, with marriage and family on the horizon.

It was apparent to anyone who knew me then (and now) that my path would be anything but linear. I'd made peace with that, but it could be frustrating to those around me, so I appreciated that Kristen was helping without making me feel pressured or undervalued. I checked out Montreat College and found that it was a small Christian school located in the mountains near a town called Black Mountain, not too far from Asheville.

I immediately loved the rugged setting surrounded by beautiful mountains, and I was intrigued by this small Christian school. My faith was relatively new, and it was much more organic and personal, not a result of scholarly study and an ability to quote Scripture upon request. I wasn't exactly sure what was expected of me as a student at a Christian college, but I called and talked to the director of the elementary education program.

"Why don't you visit us, and we can talk about it?" she said in a kind voice.

We hit it off right away. Having lost my mom a few years back, I was clearly rough around the edges and felt a connection with her.

"I love your story and your spirit," she told me. "We want our students to be happy here, and I think you'd be a great fit. Why don't you visit the school chapel today?"

I got a great vibe from her and immediately agreed. "I'd love to check it out." When I walked in, I saw that it was filled with people, so I slumped down in the back row to take it all in. The students were certainly feeling the spirit. They were singing in unison with their hands swaying in the air. I honestly wasn't sure how to feel at that moment. I'd been through a wild, rock-and-roll kind of life up to that point, and I could feel all of it coming to a screeching halt. In. That. Precise. Moment.

It was clear that I was at a fork in the road, and I wasn't sure I could pull it off. Here I was at this small Christian school with all these people praising God, but I decided to continue the journey of discovery. One of my prerequisite classes was studying the Old Testament, and I was completely lost once we began the course. I couldn't memorize the cast of characters to save my life. Which of the apostles or disciples were they talking about? Was that Paul? I could tell the other students had probably grown up studying the Bible and could recite passage and verse. When I asked questions, they looked at me like I was an alien. They were all nice enough, but they appeared to be frustrated by my elementary questions. I learned to just keep my mouth shut and take it all in.

Our teacher was my saving grace because I connected with him, and I'm sure he saw in me a guy who needed some guidance. I went up to him after class one day and said, "As you can tell, I have a long way to go with this theology stuff and understanding the history of Christianity, but I can promise you that I am interested in it. I could really use some help with the basics so that I don't feel so lost, though."

He was supportive in that class, and most of the other teachers were as well. There were a few tough ones, though. One of them was very "by the book," and he seemed a bit frustrated by my unconventional approach. During one of our sessions, he asked, "Are you excited to be here at Montreat?"

It took me by surprise. "Oh my God, yes, you have no idea how excited I am!"

"Pete, do you know you're actually using the Lord's name in vain any time you use God's name like that?" Instantly, I was embarrassed. "I just want you to understand the impact of the words you use." Well, fuck!

It was a humbling experience, but something I'd become accustomed to because of my more personal approach to religion and spirituality. However, after that, things started to click for me. I began to understand the foundation of my faith, and the nervousness I'd felt melted away. I was speaking confidently, bonding with the other students, and doing well in all my classes. It was a rewarding feeling to have it all come together in a structured environment. That was new to me.

As I began my concentration in elementary education, most of the core classes were made up of me and 12 or 13 Southern girls. There weren't a lot of guys focused on elementary ed. at that time. It was fine with me because I was used to making my own way and going against the grain. I managed to excel in my classes and graduate with honors. It was incredibly special when my grandmother and the rest of my family came to my graduation. They probably wanted to see it for themselves because I wasn't known for setting goals and achieving them. Being on stage, holding my diploma, was something they probably never expected from me.

I honestly wasn't sure I'd ever get to that point in my life. Being comfortable with following my own professional path originated with my mom. When I was 18, she said, "Pete, you don't have to go to college. I know you need to figure out stuff." I protested, saying that I wanted to go to school where my friends were going; and I did, but she was right. She was trying to tell me that it might not be the best choice for me. I bounced around several colleges, and never really applied myself or took them seriously.

So, finally graduating was a milestone for me. I began student teaching at a small private school called Asheville Christian Academy. The headmaster hired me as a sixth-grade teacher and he said, "There's a female teacher already, and she is tough. She's science-oriented, very structured, and doesn't let the kids get away with anything. We're looking to you as the male role model to provide a different viewpoint."

I quickly realized that I wasn't so effective at teaching religion to a group of 12-year-olds who knew much more about religion than I ever would. However, there was another area where I was able to help. Seeing the kids interact took me back to my own experiences with bullying and being ostracized. I made a promise to myself that, if nothing else, I would make sure those kids didn't go through that. It wasn't going to happen on my watch. I wanted to be an advocate for those kids, and I was going to make sure they all realized that each of them was special with their own unique talents.

In my class, I made it clear that as far as I was concerned, no one was cooler than anyone else. It didn't matter what they looked like, where they were from, or how shy they were. We were all in it together, and I let them know that I understood what they were going through. And I did.

There's no denying that I gave everything to my students. I listened to them. I advocated for them. I valued their opinions. I honored their individualism and focused on it every day. I was determined to make a difference. When one of them told me about issues at home, I listened, gave them some advice, and promised I'd be there for them the next day.

In my zeal to make their experience the best I could, I'll admit that we probably played too many games. I took all of them outside when I could get away with it. We'd hike down to the river and skip stones. Sometimes we'd even pull out poles I'd stashed nearby and fish for a while. This was usually happening in place of my assigned tasks, which were to instruct them on English, History, and the Bible. I taught those subjects, but not as traditionally as the administration would have liked.

I loved those *Choose Your Own Adventure* books as a kid (and I basically lived my life following that strategy), so I read those books to the class, and they loved them. During parent-teacher conferences, I received many stories of how much I had inspired their children, and how their kids loved coming to my class. That was especially true of anyone who had trouble fitting in or making friends. On the other end of the spectrum were the parents whose kids were jockeying for the highest grade and focused on education. That's where I fell short. I wasn't the best educator for them.

I even pushed the envelope when it came to religion. To me, it seemed like most of the kids saw God and Jesus as cartoon characters, and I wanted them to deepen their faith beyond Bible verses and perfect test grades. I approached the headmaster and said, "I know that the movie *The Passion of the Christ* is rated R, but I was wondering if I could just show one scene from it to my class."

To my surprise, he said, "I think it'd be fine."

The next day, I looked out at the class of mostly affluent, well-dressed kids with their innocent smiles. This was my chance to really show them the other side of religion: the suffering, the agony. "All right, kids, I'm going to show you something that I want you to pay attention to." I pushed play on the video and in full color was the crucifixion scene where Jesus was being graphically beaten and humiliated. It was more realistic than I'd remembered, and it only took about 30 seconds for me to understand the error of my ways. Kids were sobbing and covering their eyes. It was intense. It was only a matter of hours before I started receiving the emails from parents.

How dare you!

What were you thinking?

I did get one email from a parent who thanked me for showing what actually happened to our Savior, but that was the minority. Most of them were electronic ambushes aimed right for my heart. Soon, I was having meetings with the headmaster and one parent after the other. Each time, I tried to calmly explain my intentions, but they were not interested in hearing them.

After those meetings, the headmaster said, "Pete, you cannot go to the river anymore. You go there much too often. You need to focus on the curriculum."

I realized the writing was on the wall. After two years, I'd reached the kids, but I'd failed to balance that with the administrative requirements. I was expected to follow the rules, and that just was not me and it never had been. So, once I decided that I was not going to go back to teaching the following year, I told the kids, "We're going to the river one last time, but we can't let anyone know. Come on, follow me." I turned around and they were lined up behind me like excited little ducklings waddling toward the water. I told them we needed to run for it, and we did. We had an amazing afternoon listening to the frogs, watching the fish jump, and staring wistfully at the soft clouds floating in the sky. It was the perfect swan song for my educational career.

I'm proud of the impact I made on those kids, and the way I shut down any kind of bullying or entitlement. It made me so happy to think that I had helped them avoid the hell I went through.

There was a girl in my class who was incredibly shy, so I was determined to help coax her out of her shell as much as possible. I called her my rock star, and we had a secret handshake that we did every day. I loved seeing her face light up because she was getting attention and enjoying it. I could see that spark inside, and it made me want to help her as much as I could. Once, I gave the students an assignment to make a funny video of themselves. The next day when they came in, the shy girl handed me her submission.

"Don't hand it to me, rock star. Put it in there and press play!"

She did, and it was the most hilarious video of her just acting crazy, a side of her the class had never seen. They went wild and showered her with compliments. Those are the moments that I cherish from the experience. Letting those kids be as authentic as possible and giving them a safe space to do so. To me, that's more valuable than any pop quiz could ever be.

On a whim, I ran my first marathon while I was still teaching. I think I was searching for my next challenge. I came into class that Monday and shared with them that I'd been running that weekend and it was amazing.

The next day, a student came in and said, "My dad wanted me to ask if you've ever heard of the fifty-state marathon club."

Being a runner for less than 24 hours, I hadn't, but I was intrigued so I did some research. The goal of the club was to run 50 marathons, one in each state. I decided to challenge myself. By the time I left teaching, I'd completed about half of my goal. It felt good to put my energy into something physical, and I was able to enjoy the outdoors, which was my personal classroom every day. Focusing on those marathons helped me realize that I'd been trying to fit teaching into my lifestyle by taking the kids outdoors. Being inside a school all day was not where I wanted to spend my life.

Fortunately, Kristen was understanding and supportive because she knew that's what I loved doing. I also talked to my grandmother and my uncle to get their advice. After Mom and Grandpa Dobson passed away, Grandma and I became even closer. The loss we shared helped deepen our connection, and I treasured it. I was eager to get her perspective on my latest dreams and passions. She was never judgmental or dismissive of my free-spirited nature; in fact, she encouraged it.

I was clearly passionate about running and outdoor activities, so I decided it made sense to open my own running store. It would be perfect because I could promote something that I was devoted to. I'd been able to make a difference in the lives of those kids, and I could do the same for everyone by promoting physical fitness and selling running gear.

Now, I can say from experience that just because you have a passion for something like running does not mean you are qualified to own, manage, and staff a retail store. I was in way over my head with inventory and payroll and merchandise displays. An employee said to me, "You run this store like a lemonade stand." He was right about that. I didn't know enough to make financial projections, manage inventory, or prepare ahead for busy seasons.

Being in a mountain community, the store was a natural fit for all the outdoor enthusiasts. In the beginning, I was engaged in the process. I had boundless energy. Anytime someone walked in the door, I was ready to pounce. "Hey, how are you? Are you getting ready to run? Are you training for a race? Tell me your story." I'd listen to them sometimes for an hour or more. Just like with my students, I'd really advocate for them and do my best to set them up for success.

And then gradually I became jaded by the whole experience. I set up early morning group runs that were a great release, but after that, I was once again stuck inside while extolling the virtues of being outside. The more I talked, the more I realized that I wanted to be the customer getting suited up to go for a run. People would come in, and I'd spend a long time educating them on the right shoe and the best size for them. Then they'd ask me to write it down so they wouldn't forget. I realized they were going online and buying what I'd recommended. It was incredibly frustrating.

One day, a lady came in and said she'd been at my buddy's running store recently. She confessed that she'd bought three pairs of shoes from him and returned each one because they "weren't right". She was hoping I could help. I was thinking, *oh shit, she's going to do the same to me. Then I'll have to write that off because I can't return worn shoes.* Still, I said, "I'm going to take the time to fit you. I'm totally confident in my skills."

I went through the entire process with her. It took over an hour to get her situated in a great pair of shoes that she liked. She was ecstatic and said they were perfect. I was happy that I'd helped her out and probably made her into a repeat customer. Win-win. A week later, she was at my door with the box of shoes in her hand. "Pete, I thought these were the ones for me, but I started running a couple of times and I got this weird spot on my foot." Reluctantly, I said I'd see what I could do. I found her another pair and said that was it.

One week later, she was back, again with the shoes still on her feet claiming that they weren't the right shoes either. She also had her son with her. I lost my shit.

"You tried three pairs of shoes at my friend's damn place. You used all of them, gave them back to him. So he's shit outta luck. Not only that, but you come here, I fit you, you got a great pair of shoes, already returned those, and now you're bringing these back? This is bullshit, and I am done with you completely." I opened the cash register and took out $110. "Here, take this cash and leave the shoes."

"But I don't have any other shoes with me."

"Well, what did you expect if you wanted to return them?"

"So, you're sending me out of your shop barefoot?"

I said, "Hell, yeah. Get out and don't come back!"

To promote the shop, I'd gotten into social media and was generating a bit of traction for the store. Just down the street was an ice cream shop that usually had a different clientele than mine. Most of my customers were fitness oriented, and most of those at the ice cream store were not. I had put a bench right outside of my place for people to switch into their new shoes if they wanted to.

One day I came to work and there were people lined up and down the street at the ice cream shop, but no one around my shop. I was super frustrated with the lack of business. Then I looked out my shop window and three ladies were parked on my bench eating ice cream even though there were seats elsewhere for that. I went out there and began sweeping around them to give them the hint that I wanted to keep the entrance-way clear. Oblivious to my actions, they continued to talk even louder. I finally asked, "Can you ladies just leave? You're sitting here eating this ice cream and that's not what I'm trying to promote in front of my running store."

They seemed taken aback but agreed to move on. I was still upset and frustrated with my lack of business, so I got on Facebook and shared my infinite wisdom with anyone who wanted to read it.

"I am sick and tired of these heifers coming to sit on my bench, eating gargantuan ice cream cones while I'm trying to inspire a community to run. I'm just tired of it."

I pressed "send" and then went to lunch. I came back two hours later and checked my post. It had over 150 comments and they were continuing to build.

You asshole, how in the hell can you say that?

You know, you're the type of person who makes people not want to come to the gym because they feel judged and feel they will never measure up.

Who do you think you are?

Then there were comments from people trying to defend me, and it kept building like a social cyclone. People were saying mean things back and forth. It was yet another sign that I had no business running a retail store and dealing with the public. Why would I ever write something like that? It was natural to get frustrated with people, but I couldn't let that interfere with my success. Customer service was obviously not something I had a handle on.

It got to the point where I got annoyed when someone opened the shop door, and the cheerful bell would ring. I started to hate that ringing bell. Toward the end of my two years there, the financial aspect was coming to a head, and again I saw the writing on the wall. It was miserable. I'd see people walking down the street enjoying the outdoors and laughing with each other while I was—again—trapped in a prison of my own making.

The final straw came when I was trying to help a lady who had wandered in. She was playing the coy game of "I'm not sure if I'm going to buy anything today." At that point, I didn't care either way. Then the phone rang. It was my brother.

"Hey, Scott, how are you?" I asked. Scott had moved to Colorado in August of 1999 to attend the University of Colorado, Boulder. After graduating, he headed to Telluride to do a little snowboard instructing and a lot of partying. He eventually landed in Kauai, Hawaii, with his girlfriend, but he couldn't resist the stronghold that Colorado has on the Ripmasters, and he eventually settled there with his family. Dad instilled two things in all of us—a love for sports and an appreciation for the West.

"Pete, you know how we always used to wonder what rock bottom was going to be for Dad?"

"Yeah, of course." No matter where I was traveling or living, Scott was always good about keeping me updated on family drama. He was at home when Dad fell through the shower door. Scott said he heard a huge crash and Mom's scream slice through the early morning calm. After a night of shenanigans on one of his sales trips, Dad had come home and hopped in the shower. After he got out, he was peeing in the toilet when he passed out and fell backward. Somehow, he managed to smash his head through the glass shower door, his body splayed on the bathroom floor and blood everywhere. Scott helped ease him away from the glass until the paramedics arrived. The man had a way of cheating death, until he didn't.

"Well, you don't need to worry about Dad anymore."

"What do you mean?"

"Dad died last night. He drove off a cliff outside of Telluride and died on impact."

I hung up the phone and sat down. I couldn't move. I didn't know what to do. Just the night before, I had taken Kristen to a Merle Haggard concert. I had a chance to meet my musical hero and sit backstage at his show. It was one of the best nights of my life. Now, the very next day, I was getting the news that my dad was dead.

Meanwhile, my customer said she wanted to buy the shoes.

"I'm sorry," I told her. "You have to go. I'm closing. I have something going on, and I need you to leave."

I locked the door and fell onto my couch. There was a decorative tree in the middle of the store, and I watched as one of the old, dusty leaves came loose and slowly drifted to the ground. Once it landed, I started crying and gasping to catch my breath. I couldn't believe I'd lost my dad.

Chapter Nine

Re-Trail Therapy

The goal to run 50 marathons did not come out of left field, but I know it seemed that way. In the fall of 2008, I had just taken my grandmother and sister to the airport so they could catch a flight home after their visit to Asheville. Once they were out of the car, I turned to my wife and said, "You know, today's the day I'm going to run a marathon," and then I pulled away from the curb.

Because we'd been together for a while, Kristen was used to my way of thinking and communicating. It was not unlike me to make a declaration that she had no idea was under consideration. Of course, anything that I committed to was something I'd been contemplating internally. That's the way I've always been—more interior and self-reflective than people might realize. It's true that I'm a what-you-see-is-what-you-get kind of guy, but there's also the other side. Since I was a kid, I'd retreat into myself and think things over, sometimes to the point of obsession. After I'd examined an issue from every angle, I was then ready to make a decision and see it through.

When I made that running declaration, Kristen looked over at all 6'1" and 230 pounds of me and said, "Where is that coming from?" I knew she would be supportive of whatever I decided, but I wasn't sure if she realized how serious I was.

At that point, I looked more like a former linebacker who hadn't stepped on the field in years than a marathon runner. My lifestyle was centered around drinking and eating junk food. To be clear, I was jolly. A big boy. I had no trouble cleaning my plate at every meal. In fact, when I look back at some pictures from that time, I often had some type of food in my hand. I couldn't be bothered to set it down for a photo.

Kristen and I had been married for a couple of years by then, and I was well into my "let it go" period while she continued to focus on her fitness. She's been a vegetarian most of her life and follows a disciplined workout regimen. She doesn't deviate no matter what. It's impressive and inspiring, and yet I was the opposite. We were a before-and-after couple. I appreciated that she never made me feel like I was making bad choices. Instead, her approach was to show me what smart, healthy choices looked like.

It's funny how certain memories stick in our brains. I clearly remember the point of no return. One day, while I was at a gym in downtown Asheville, idly jogging on the treadmill in a half-hearted attempt to jumpstart my fitness, I looked out the window and saw that traffic was at a standstill. In one car, I saw a man reading a newspaper and eating fast food that was balanced on his stomach along with his cell phone. I shuddered and thought, *Oh, my gosh, that's what giving up in middle age looks like!* Then I cranked up the speed on the treadmill and was on my way.

For my first attempt at a marathon, I asked Kristen to drive me to the Blue Ridge Parkway and drop me off. I knew they had mile markers and thought that would be a start. I was wearing old Nike tennis shoes , cotton socks, cotton boxers, cargo shorts, a cotton shirt, a fleece vest, and a camo hat. Definitely not the best running gear, but I didn't know any better.

Kristen drove ahead of me to begin strategically placing power bars and sports drinks at every third mile. I started jogging in the same direction, planning to run 13.1 miles—the distance equal to half a marathon—and then double back to complete the challenge. After just a couple of minutes, though, I saw her driving back toward me.

"The parkway is closed right around the corner. The gates are down so no cars can get around it," she said.

"Oh," I said. "Well, I'm going anyway. I'm doing this today. Just hand me the biggest Gatorade we've got, and I'll carry it."

I ran around the gate, onto the parkway, and then realized I was running *up* the mountain. It was 13.1 miles straight up towards Mt. Pisgah, but I didn't stop. I basically waddled the entire way. Once I miraculously reached the top at 13.1 miles, I started back down. Kristen was waiting for me at the gate, which I finally reached although I was puffing and wheezing the entire time. I still had to go another 1.2 miles to complete the distance, so I told her that I would meet her at the bottom of the hill.

That 1.2 miles took me almost half an hour to complete, and I was a mess at the end of it. I was sweating, gasping for air, my thighs were sore from rubbing together, and the old shoes irritated my feet. I laid down and was hot one second and cold the next. I felt like I was going to either throw up or worse, but I didn't. Despite all that discomfort, I had done it! I'd finished! When Kristen drove up, I pulled myself into the car and smiled. "I love this!" I said. It was clear to me that I *needed* to run.

I was still teaching at the time, and the following Monday, I told my class what I had done. That's when one of the students told me about the 50 marathons in 50 states club. That night I was on the computer checking out their website, and I saw that sometimes the runner raised money for a cause while running the states. That's when the pieces came together. I could take on this challenge and raise money for cancer research in my mom's name—something I had promised her I'd do before she died. I would run 50 marathons in 50 states by the time I was 50 with a goal of raising $50,000. It felt like a sign, an indication that this was meant to be.

Even though I hadn't played sports for a while, I was still in my 30s and my athletic physique started coming back, slowly but surely. Changing my eating habits was paying off. I also began fundraising for the charity, and the dollars started rolling in. I was on my way!

There was a definite learning curve. I completed roughly 12 marathons a year and never trained between them. I had a solid jog for half of the marathon and somewhere around the 16th mile, I'd hit a wall. Still, I didn't stop. I'd shuffle, slow jog, walk, whatever I had to do to finish, as everyone else ran past me.

My 30th race was in the northeast, and just like the others, I started out with a good run before hitting a wall. I watched everyone sail past—many older than me, some with physical challenges. That's when I realized that while I was committed to the goal, I wasn't fully invested. Between marathons, I needed to put in the work. It wasn't enough for me to just go through the motions.

So, I started a training program, and that's when I opened the running shop. It became a lifestyle. I trained for two hours in the morning and then opened the store at 10 a.m. I talked running all day, then hopefully got in a little run after closing. I also started a running group, and we trained together. My marathon finishing times went from five-and-a-half hours down to four. Then, during a dream run that comes around once in a blue moon, I looked at my watch and realized I was close to breaking three hours and actually had a good chance at qualifying for the prestigious Boston Marathon. (That marathon is notoriously difficult to get in. You need a time nearly five minutes faster than your age requirement and the set standard for your gender.) For my run, I fell off a bit at the end but still ran 3:05, easily qualifying for Boston.

Somewhere during my self-imposed challenge to complete 50 marathons in 50 states, my runs morphed into internal therapy sessions. Each one started out basically the same. In the beginning, I was solely focused on the physicality of it all—the weather, my body, the terrain—but before I realized what was happening, my mind began to wander. I would reel myself back and return my focus to the run; but it would happen again—thoughts jockeying for my attention, a wheel of emotions spinning around before finally landing. What would it be this time? Pride? Confidence? Arrogance? Doubt? Fear? Sorrow?

During one of those marathons, I was in New Jersey running a trail that had a loop as part of the course. It was the middle of winter, and the weather was brutal. Mentally, the spinning wheel had landed on self-pity and doubt. I was questioning myself and my abilities. That's not helpful when I'm in the middle of a tough course. My pace was slowing, and I felt beaten down. It was just one of those days.

This course was a little different because it had a cutoff time. Runners had to arrive at the designated aid station before it was too late. After that, the station would close, and any latecomers would not be recognized as official finishers. For me, that would mean repeating the race another year. I'd already had a bad morning and arrived late, but I convinced them to let me join the run because I was nearing my 50-state goal. However, things weren't looking good. This was not one of those perfect races where everything aligned. This time, the combination of the bad weather, my late arrival, and nagging self-doubt was negatively affecting my performance.

I reached a fork in the trail and came to a stop. I realized that I had been on the loop twice already. I'd have to run a wide circle for another several miles and then curve back around.

Looking down, I saw that it would be easy to cut through the woods and get back on the course, and that would shave a few miles off so that I could finish on time. No one was around, so what would it hurt? I already knew that I could run the course. They knew I could do it, my supporters and donors knew I could do it, so what would be the big deal? It would make things so much easier.

Long-distance running tests us physically, but it's the mental fitness that really comes into play. It's not just putting on tennis shoes and jogging a few miles. It's an intense, immersive experience that puts you to the test. The questions are, will you pass, and will you be proud of yourself? That's one of the reasons why running fulfills me in ways that a college degree or a traditional job never could. I like to put myself in difficult situations and make choices that I'm proud of.

Clearly, I could never cheat on my run because it would go against everything I stand for. When I was weaker and less confident, things may have turned out differently, but I'd worked hard to improve my physical and mental growth. There was zero chance that I'd jeopardize that no matter how beneficial it might be. So, I dutifully turned left and continued on that damn loop that had tempted and taunted me. I was happy with my decision, but that didn't change the fact that I was exhausted, I didn't like the course, and I wanted it to be over.

Another aspect of running that I love is sharing it with others and watching them get excited about it. When I first started my marathon journey, I gave Scott a call and told him about it, and how I was raising money in Mom's name.

"That's amazing, Pete," he said. "Kudos to you, man. I think it's an awesome idea and I'll donate, but I want nothing else to do with it."

"Well," I told him, "I'd like you to run one with me."

"I might crew for you, but that's a foolish distance. I just don't have time for it."

"Scott, I'm committed to doing 50 of them. You hear me? Five-oh. I think you can do one." I knew he wouldn't let me down.

"OK, man, I'll do a marathon with you."

I was pumped. "Great! Look at a map, pick a state that I haven't done yet, and we're on!"

Of course, Scott picked Alaska, arguably the most challenging terrain, but I was down. I even gave him a training program to follow so he could prepare. He ended up running more than a few marathons with me and having him as a part of it makes them even more special for me.

Haig seemed surprised when I told him about the 50 marathons; but of course, he was supportive. "You know, it's mostly mental," he said. "You've got more mental strength than anybody I know. I'm sure you can do it. You have to unlock that ability and push through the pain." He even joined me on marathon runs in Oregon and Colorado. Colorado was my last marathon in the project, and I went out with a bang. I had Asleep at the Wheel, my favorite band, play the finish party with nearly 100 friends and family there to celebrate with me. Yee Haw!

Running has taught me that there is nothing wrong with questioning yourself. I was used to doing that. What could I have done to help my mom fight cancer? Could I have stopped Dad from his self-destructive behavior? Why didn't teaching satisfy me? How could I screw up a successful running store? Those thoughts used to come at me hard and fast. Meeting Kristen was one of the best things that ever happened to me. The other was discovering my love for running. The reassurance I got from her, matched with the confidence I learned from running, helped piece my puzzling life together. Things began to fall into place, to make sense, and to fulfill me like never before.

One of my running tricks is to stop the negative thoughts before they have a chance to derail my focus. When I'm 12 miles in on a marathon with 14.2 left to go, that's when a strong mind is challenged. So, at the first hint of negativity, I shift the focus to numbers. They are easy for me to wrap my mind around because they are steadfast, unyielding. They either are or they aren't. There's no second-guessing. No room for doubt. *A marathon is 26.2 miles. I round it up to 27 miles. That's nine three-mile runs, which is nine 5Ks. That's doable. Of course, I can do that!*

Courses in big cities often have the mile markers along the road which makes it even easier for me to break it down into manageable chunks. *OK, I've got to get myself to that first three-mile marker. I'm one 5K into this marathon.* Sometimes, I actually hold out my hand, look at it, fold in my thumb and three fingers with only the forefinger extended and think, *that's one!* It's a physical reminder that I can refer to so that I don't lose focus.

Next, I think about getting from mile three to mile six. I never focus on the fact that I'm 25% of the way to 26.2 miles. I keep it in three-mile sections, which to me signifies a local run that I do at home all the time. I just have to do those four more times to finish the marathon etc.

Then, when I'm on the last one, there are only 2.2 miles left because I rounded up. The ninth 5K is only 2.2 miles! So next thing I know, I feel my hands tighten and look down to see that I've been counting three-mile increments on my hand without even realizing it. And then, I'm turning the corner and the finish line is in sight. I nailed the run! Some athletes I've shared that with think it's a strange way to run, but it's what works for me. I've learned over the years to trust my instincts even though my methods may not make sense to anyone else.

Another thing I practice is the art of allowing myself a lot of grace when I'm running. Graduating from trails to multiple marathons meant I had to become comfortable with my method and allow it to lead me to the finish line. As a result, it has given me a better understanding of who I am. It has opened me up to a level of mindfulness that I would have never known otherwise. What I discovered was that I need to run. It's something I no longer take for granted. Finding my purpose helped me reach personal goals and even allowed me to give back. Through my goal of running 50 marathons in 50 states, I raised over $62,000 for cancer research in just five years.

As with my journey in life, my running journey has not been linear or traditional. I went from personal trail runs to surviving the wilds of Alaska to running marathons across the country. My next personal challenge was moving into the world of ultramarathons, which was totally different from anything I had experienced before.

Ultramarathons are typically anything beyond a traditional 26.2-mile marathon. So technically, running 50 kilometers, which is a little more than 31 miles, is an ultramarathon. It's basically semantics because just running a few more miles more than a marathon means that someone can call themselves an ultramarathon runner. I've never understood that.

When I first heard about the ultras, I was in Oklahoma finishing up a trail marathon. As I was heading back to my hotel room, I saw the gym with a treadmill in it. I thought, *this is it! I'm going to run my first ultra.* After picking up my marathon finisher medal, I was in the hotel workout room running 5 extra miles so I could be a 50K finisher! It was a pretty weak first ultra, but I put in the work and stuck to it. In no time, I was running a double marathon in the Rocky Mountains. It was either a 26.2-mile marathon or a double marathon at 52.4 miles. You finish the marathon, then you turn around and do the exact same route again, so it ends up being a 52.4-miles—a true ultra. My brother happened to be there at the time and ran with me, which again made it even more special.

One thing I discovered was that I really benefited from the mental challenge as well as the physical. My experience in rock climbing and mountaineering definitely came into play and helped me push through those tough mountain trails. I knew that's what I was born to do, and I began to realize why I never successfully applied myself in team sports at school. That just wasn't my passion. I preferred to do it all myself; that way I knew that any success I had was well-earned. There was no one to rely on except me.

Soon, I completed my first hundred-mile race. Those races mean running nonstop, through the night, and can take anywhere from 20 to 40 hours to complete. Typically, runners carry a backpack with spare clothes, food, and drink because aid stations are spaced extremely far apart.

Conquering each challenge was a building block in not only my running career but my self-confidence. I couldn't believe that with training and willpower, I was able to run 100 miles with my own two feet! That was amazing to me, and it had happened organically as I became a more experienced runner.

One day in 2013, I was reading *Ultrarunning Magazine* (because that's what we ultrarunners do) when I saw an article about the Iditarod Trail Invitational. Alaska still held a special place in my heart, so I was curious about what the article described as "the world's longest winter ultramarathon and one of the most challenging experiences on the planet."

How in the hell did I not know about this? Was it going on while I was hunkered down in my Alaskan cabin? Of course, I'd heard about the traditional Iditarod, the famed dog sled race, but the Trail Invitational was different. It was a race made up of runners, bikers, and skiers—human power as opposed to dog power. I read the article and immediately thought, *this is me! I need to be a part of this race!*

The ITI is the longest winter ultramarathon and considered the ultimate personal physical challenge. The trail winds through rugged Alaska mountain ranges without ever crossing a road. It's remote, raw, and rugged. No doubt it's the holy grail of extreme sports, and I couldn't stop thinking about it. There would be no aid stations and no crowds cheering me on. It would be the ultimate challenge and a true test of the skills I'd amassed over the past several years.

I quickly emailed the ITI race director to find out how I could be a part of this amazing experience. I extolled my accomplishments, mentioned the 50 marathons, and assured him I was up for the challenge.

"I need to run this race. I've spent years of my life in Alaska and am interested in running the ITI 350. I don't know how else to say this, but I have to run this race. Please respond when you have a chance. I'm really looking forward to hearing back from you."

Of course, as usual, I also had included a risqué quote from Yvon Chouinard, an American rock climber, environmentalist, and businessman who is the founder of the Patagonia brand:

"Taking a trip for six months, you get in the rhythm of it. It feels like you can go on forever doing that. Climbing Everest is the ultimate and the opposite of that. Because you get these high-powered plastic surgeons and CEOs and, you know, they pay $80,000 and have Sherpas put the ladders in place and 8,000 feet of fixed ropes and you get to the camp, and you don't even have to lay out your sleeping bag. It's already laid out with a chocolate mint on the top. The whole purpose of planning something like Everest is to effect some sort of spiritual and physical gain, and if you compromise the process, you're an asshole when you start out and you're an asshole when you get back."

I was ecstatic when the race director wrote back, although he basically said that I was either truly motivated or a potential nut case. He also pointed out that running marathons didn't mean much when it came to the ITI; however, he did like that I had lived in the Alaskan wilderness, and he was very impressed by the quote I'd sent along! His last few words were something I'll never forget. "Without the journey, the destination is worthless."

I hadn't run a single qualifier, but he invited me to sign up anyway. He was willing to take a chance on me, and I couldn't have been happier. I trained as much as I could even though I didn't really know what I was doing. I had no idea what I was getting myself into. I'd never done 350 miles in such a brutal climate. I had no clue.

However, I had fallen into a comfortable rhythm where physical challenges were concerned. I'd conquer one goal, then find another and work hard until I crushed that one, too. Somehow, over the years I'd learned to channel that cockiness and natural athletic ability of my youth into constructive, fulfilling, positive motivation that allowed me to meet each challenge head-on.

In just a few short years, I'd toughed out the Alaskan wilderness, excelled at marathons, and tackled ultramarathons. Each time, I learned more about myself and further confirmed that I was following God's plan for me. The frustration I'd felt trying to fit into team sports and societal molds of traditional careers melted away when I was on a run. It was clear to me that I'd found my niche, my place in this world.

I couldn't have been more amped to get back to the Alaskan wilderness and prove my mettle. I had already put my body and mind to the test time and again. It was amazing to look at how far I'd come in just a few short years. Channeling my frustrations and focusing on physical goals had provided the personal satisfaction that had eluded me for so long. The only thing that would have made the journey even sweeter would have been if my parents were still alive; but I know they would have been so happy that I had finally found my true purpose.

Chapter Ten

Choose Your Own Adventure

I couldn't believe that not only was I going to take part in the ITI, but that I'd also be back in the 49th state. It would be yet another physical challenge on my journey to explore ultramarathons. While I was familiar with the unforgiving region, I knew practically nothing about the event, and there wasn't a lot of information to be found. There were plenty of stories about the traditional dog sled race; however, the ITI was something of a mystery. Still, I was curious and fixated on my next adventure.

Fortunately, I was able to talk with an elite athlete from Colorado who had recently finished the 350-mile race. He was a well-known ultra-runner in our small circles, and he was one of the few who had competed in the ITI on foot (as opposed to bikes or skis). I shot rapid-fire questions at him, and he gave me lots of feedback and even shared a copy of his gear list. Apparently, the things you pack can either make or break your experience on the trail.

I continued searching for other participants to find out what they took with them. I was on a fact-finding mission.

Packing was an art of its own because the gear had to be useful for survival, beneficial for athletic performance, and light enough to transport over 350 miles of mountainous terrain.

One of the celebrated athletes who had finished the ITI in first place several times is a wild man named Dave Johnston. He's a North Carolina boy living in Alaska with his awesome family. Dave's got a long blonde ponytail, a laid-back attitude, and an easy smile. Since we were both from N.C., I decided to reach out to him and get his input on my attempt at the race. I wasn't sure he'd respond, but I sure was excited when he did. He was amazingly gracious and even agreed to meet up with me before my first Iditarod Trail Invitational. Awesome!

In February of 2014, 50 invited participants from around the world gathered in Anchorage to begin the race. Most of us were competing in the 350-mile journey that stretched over the Alaska Range leading to McGrath. However, some of the competitors were going all the way to Nome, for a total of 1,000 miles. Getting to McGrath was enough of a challenge for me as a newbie.

Arriving in Anchorage, I was like a deer in the headlights. I wasn't sure what I was getting into, but I was pumped to get started. I was so stoked, and a little star struck when Dave dropped by my hotel room with his son in tow. It was exciting stuff for an up-and-coming athlete, but I tried to stay cool and focus on the race the next day.

"How are you doing, man?" he asked me. "You all set for tomorrow?"

"I'm ready! I have my checklist, and my gear is ready," I replied.

"OK," he said. "I'm happy to help rookies out, so I'll check your sled weight if you want."

Once outside, I went over to my sled, and he followed. Then he grabbed it with one hand, but it wouldn't budge. He couldn't lift it! He tried again by holding it with the straps and getting more leverage, but it was useless. All he said was, "Yeah, that seems about right."

He was too nice to say that I had screwed myself. He didn't want to scare me because there wasn't much that I could do about it at that point. I'd thrown in everything I could think of to make sure I was covered for any situation. That meant that I was saddled with more weight than I should have been to successfully navigate the perilous trail. They say you carry all your insecurities with you on your first ITI adventure. They were right.

I went down to the lobby the next morning and found myself among a group of elite athletes. The energy was palpable, and I could hardly believe that I'd managed to break into this club. Some of the folks seemed very sure of themselves and somewhat standoffish, which was fine. I wasn't there to make friends. This was a personal challenge for me. I went off to the side by myself to calm my nerves and prepare for the journey that was about to take place.

"Hey everyone," a voice bellowed, "there is a scale over there. Let's line up and weigh our sleds before we get started." Remember, the foot athletes haul a sled behind them.

I watched guys and gals pull their sleds onto the scale. With the first sled on the scale, the racer closest to the scale said, "OK, 41 pounds."

The racer seemed dejected. "I didn't want it to be over 40. I'm gonna take something out."

I was standing in the back of the room with my mouth hanging open. These guys were hardcore and obsessing over one pound. The only thing I could focus on were the numbers I was hearing:

"35!"

"32!"

"30 pounds!"

Please make it stop. This was not going to end well. I already knew that I was maxed out after Dave tried to lift my gear, so I started to back up slowly. I could just skip this part. Who would know?

"OK, Ripmaster, bring your sled over here."

That stopped me in my tracks. "Oh, no, man, don't worry about it," I said. "I'm good."

Before I knew it, two guys came over, took my sled, and dragged it up front. My heart began to race, my mind was spinning. I'd basically weaseled my way into the race, was trying to impress the other competitors, and didn't want to look like some kind of rookie who couldn't pack a sled. As long as I wasn't too much over 40 pounds, I could probably just laugh it off and yank something out before I got started.

There was a crowd around the scale like it was a roulette wheel and they were cheering on their lucky numbers. Once they hoisted my sled up, everyone took a step back and stared at the dial as it went past 20, 30, 35, 40. I could hear murmurs in the crowd. Then it went past 50. "Wow," someone whispered, but we weren't done. The digits continued to whirl past 60 and 70. "Holy shit," I heard from some dude to my left. I could feel my face getting flushed as the scale finally settled on a number—92. I was going to be dragging 92 pounds along a rough, primitive trail for 350 freaking miles!

The fellow racer paused for what seemed like an eternity before he said, "Ripmaster, what the hell do you have in there?" Everyone broke out in laugher as I tried to make myself invisible. "Seriously, Ripmaster, what's in there, a Coleman stove?"

"Well, uhh, I..." What could I say? There was no way for me to save face, and the entire room was still laughing and shaking their heads in disbelief. I tried to pull it off as best I could. "OK, OK, I get it. It's a lot, but it is what it is. I'm comfortable with what I've packed, and I'm excited to get started." With my sled more than double the weight of any others, I followed the group out to the bus that would take us to the starting line.

As we were getting ready to start, a legend who had completed the course many times helped tie my poles to my harness. That's when I realized just how much I was in over my head. Physical challenges had often come easily for me and running marathons gave me the confidence that this race would be similar. So, I hadn't trained by pulling a sled, hadn't learned how to pack, and couldn't tie my poles to my harness. This made me question my abilities, which is not a productive use of time just before an event is about to start.

After taking just a few steps, I realized exactly how heavy 92 pounds was when being pulled behind you in the snow. On the first little dip in the trail, my sled had so much momentum that it practically ran me over. I ended up on my ass with my poles twisted and the sled leading the way. That happened many, many more times on the trail. Sometimes, it even flipped over. It was a mess, and that was before we even began.

We all made our way down to the starting line at the lake. Tyrell Seavey, a friend of mine from my brief dog mushing days came out to see me off. "Hey, let me take some pictures of you before you get started," he said.

I wasn't keen on having any reminders of this disaster. "Oh, I appreciate that, but I'm good, man. I just want to get going." Despite my objections, he did get one photo. In most pictures from the starting line, the racers are serious, intense, and focused on the brutal event that lies ahead. In my photo, I was grinning like a clueless schoolkid, poles in hand (because they kept coming loose), and an oversized sled taunting me in the background.

Once it started, everyone was eager to get down the trail. I started out slow and steady. Not long after the start, we had to cross a frozen lake and head uphill. I was already sweating profusely as I stabbed each pole into the ground to pull myself up the trail at a snail's pace. I would take one step and get pulled back two. Every muscle in my legs ached and my arms began to burn with pain.

Some guys had unfortunately found themselves behind my slow ass, and they couldn't contain their frustration. I could hear them over my labored breathing.

"What the hell is this guy doing?"

"He has no idea what he got into."

"Come on, man, this is hard to watch!"

I was tired, frustrated, and embarrassed. "Just fucking leave me alone!" I yelled over my shoulder as I finally, miraculously, reached the top of the hill. This was just the beginning of the trail, and I felt like I'd already maxed out my energy. I wanted to turn back. It was clear to me and everyone else that I was not ready for this extreme challenge.

Somehow, I managed to keep going. About six miles in, I decided to practice with the fancy oversized GPS that I'd bought since I hadn't bothered to familiarize myself with it before the event. How hard could it be? I turned it on and saw the green light flash, but I had no idea how to program it. I shoved it in my pocket and kept moving, looking at it occasionally hoping for an alert if I went off-track. Somehow, I missed a turn or overlooked a sign and ended up 12½ miles in the wrong direction, on a frozen body of water, and it was getting late.

Even if I wanted to, I didn't know how to retrace my steps back to the starting line. I couldn't see any other racers or hear any voices since I was so far off the trail. The only saving grace I had was that monstrous pack of gear. There were enough supplies to sustain me for a long time, so I decided to set up camp on that frozen lake because I couldn't go much farther without rest.

My brand-new sleeping bag was cozy, and I had everything I needed, but I couldn't relax. I couldn't stop replaying the day's events over and over in my head. While not even close to the same scale, the negative comments and low-key hostility from the others pulled me right back to that lonely time when I was ostracized as a kid. Those feelings made me question every-thing and that undermined my one true strength—confidence. Not just confidence in myself, but always trying to stay in a positive frame of mind. Things will work out. I will figure it out. I always have.

But this time felt different.

What was I thinking? Why had I placed so much emphasis on getting accepted to the ITI and so little on preparation? Of course, I would have gone back and changed things if I could have, but I'd gotten myself into a situation that I needed to fig-ure out. There's an old saying that I try to live by in difficult times: improvise, adapt, overcome. I decided to focus on the problem and think it through logically while putting aside the gamut of emotions I'd experienced in the past 24 hours.

I knew that I was supposed to be heading northwest and that I wasn't. To make matters worse, there were snowmobiles headed every which way to further confuse me. I finally found what seemed like a promising trail heading in the correct di-rection, but that only brought me back to a spot I had already been. I was enraged. It was obvious to me now that I had headed north much sooner than I should've. That was a rookie error, but I didn't need to beat myself up about it. I was fo-cused on a solution. All other racers were at least 50 miles ahead of me by that point, so it wasn't like someone might come by later.

Either I could quit and find my way back to the start line with my tail between my legs or I could keep moving, turn northwest, and try to find the original trail. I had about 345 miles to go, and since I'd stopped so early, I probably wouldn't see anyone else until I got to the end. If I continued, I'd be alone the entire time. Somehow, I was able to calm my racing thoughts and get a little sleep.

The next morning, I felt like I'd had a mental reset. With my ego intact, I felt confident that I could improvise, adapt, and overcome my situation. At that moment, I looked ahead and could see light reflecting off what looked like one of the trail maps in a wood frame that dotted the wilderness. The sun was bouncing off the glass, and it was definitely a sign of hope.

I made my way over to study the old map, but I couldn't find a location marker anywhere. That didn't do me any good because it was impossible to determine where I was based on the nondescript landscape. I decided to go a bit farther and ran into another map. That one was more worn, but it had exactly what I needed—a marker that indicated my current location.

OK, I thought, *I can do this. If I take this trail to that trail, it will get me back on track.* It was as plain as day, and that gave me the motivation I needed. Soon, I was on the right trail and pulling my huge sled after going 25+ miles out of my way. Then it began to snow. Great. I had snowshoes in the back of my sled, but I was wearing boots with spikes on the bottom to help with traction on the ice and snow. I got the idea to combine the two and slipped my cleated running shoes into the snowshoe binding. I'd never worn snowshoes before, so I mistakenly made the binding as tight as possible. I went about two miles over treacherous terrain when both of my feet started to feel hot, like they were burning. What the hell was going on? Then I felt pain and realized I'd cinched the snowshoes so tight that the spikes were going through my insoles and into the bottom of my feet. It felt like I was standing on the sharp end of 200 golf tees.

That meant I had no choice but to stop and take off my shoes. I thought there would be a lot of punctures in my feet, but instead, they had started to blister from heel to toe. I was only one full day into the race, and I could barely walk. The pain was excruciating. My solution was to balance on my heels to relieve the pressure from the rest of my foot while still pulling a 92-pound sled.

Something kept motivating me to move forward. I don't know if it was courage, ego, determination, or sheer stupidity. I kept going, and against all odds reached the first checkpoint, 59 miles into the race. I might as well have climbed Mt. Everest after what I'd been through.

I saw the rustic Yentna Station Roadhouse dwarfed by tall trees on all sides. I knew I was in dead last place and had a feeling all involved with the race would be incredibly happy to see me! I grabbed some gear and threw open the cabin door, excited for my first check-in. It couldn't have been two seconds before I heard, "Close the fucking door." Not quite the welcome I expected.

Heat is everything in Alaska, especially in the dead of winter. There I was, storming in like some kind of hero because there were times when I didn't think I'd make it that far. To me, it was kind of heroic. "Uh, sorry about that," I said as I quickly closed the door and realized there was no welcoming committee. As expected, everyone else who was racing had already checked in and moved on.

I took off my shoes and headed to a room upstairs to dry my gear. It was dark, and the stairs were lit with dim reflective lights. There was an extra step that I didn't compensate for and kicked with my bare foot. My big toe made a popping sound. I couldn't yell because other travelers were sleeping, so I limped to one of the rooms as my toe turned colors and the nail began to come off.

Sitting down, I took stock of the mess I was in. Only about 24 hours had passed and besides massively over packing, I'd already gotten lost and messed up my feet with almost 300 more miles to go. Not only that, but now I had a broken toe to deal with. Knowing I needed to do better, I took out my trusty Iditarod map to make sure I would go in the right direction the next morning. Sitting with a local at Yentna Station who knew the trail better than anybody around, I picked his brain.

I pointed to a penciled-in Iditarod Trail route that my friend back in N.C. had helped me with and asked about the next section. He said, "This is nice, but you do know that the trail comes in different every single year, right? You know that, right?"

"Oh, yeah, of course," I said. I didn't know that, but I was so glad he helped me out because now I had the correct trail so that I could start fresh in the morning. After a decent night's sleep, I felt confident and energized, so I pushed on, following my new trusty map to make sure I didn't stray off the trail. Once I reached the next checkpoint, about 90 miles in, I was greeted with the nickname "Red Lantern."

Lanterns have a long history in the Iditarod. Every year, the committee hangs one on the arch at the end of the race in Nome and it remains lit until the final musher reaches the finish line. It's referred to as the Widow's Lamp and symbolizes the days of the Gold Rush when dogsleds were used to transport mail and other goods through the snow and darkness, often lit only with kerosene lamps outside rustic stores and taverns along the way.

The Red Lantern Award came about in the 1950s as a name for the dogsled racer who came in last place in the Iditarod. It's meant as a term of endearment and a way to celebrate an incredible achievement, even if it is for last place. It's about perseverance and personal triumph, which is as well-earned as a first-place ribbon.

There was no doubt that I was in last place, but I sure as hell didn't like to be reminded of that fact. I thought, *that's the worst title I've ever heard*. I understood that it was not meant maliciously, but I'm a lifetime competitor and athlete. Don't count me out just yet.

A woman took my picture and posted it on Facebook along with the update: *The Red Lantern has arrived!* I saw the post and wasn't happy about it. My family and friends seemed excited, and they were making supportive comments like, "There's Pete!" "He's really doing it!" and, "Go Pete!" With my unwelcomed moniker and a boost from those comments, I was back out on the trail and fighting the snow and ice.

One night while sleeping on the trail, I'd readjusted and somehow my arm ended up outside of my sleeping bag and rested in the snow for hours. I woke up and couldn't feel a thing. I used my other hand to bring it inside to examine for frostbite. I didn't see any discoloration, so I spent the next hour or so massaging and warming my arm to get the feeling back. Without it, I couldn't unzip my bag or tie my shoes, or anything.

It was truly a scary moment because nothing was happening, and I was worried about the long-term effects. I started to blame myself, but then remembered that no matter how careful someone is, nature is unpredictable, and everything can't be planned out. I was worried that I'd have to be rescued, which scared me because going out on my own terms was one thing but having to tap out because of something like this would be tough to handle.

There was one point where I felt my mind could unravel, and I was actually arguing with someone else, "No, that's not helping. Move it this way. Use the hand warmers. How's that? Any better?"

Then I said, "No, it's not working! What's wrong with you?" I turned to face an adversary that didn't exist. When I realized I was yelling at an ice-covered fir tree, I figured I was losing my mind. There was no one for miles and miles, and here I was yelling at a freakin' tree about my jacked-up arm.

I thought, *OK, Pete, get it together. Get back on the trail, get moving, make sure you're going the right way. You need some help; you're starting to unravel, dude. Come on!*

Moments like that float to the top of my brain sometimes as a reminder of how fragile and delicate my mind can be. Maybe that was a coping mechanism or just a cry for help. I'm not sure, but I do know that I learned a lot from that experience about my personal strengths and weaknesses.

Others have shared similar stories about being out in the wilderness when their mind seemed to lose its grip on reality and false perceptions took over. It's a type of panoramic hallucination exacerbated by the extreme surroundings. I suppose it's like being in the desert, another extreme climate, and hearing or seeing things that aren't actually there. It's an interesting and enlightening experience that can teach you a lot about yourself.

Somehow, I made it to the mile 200 checkpoint, and the race director was there.

"How are you doing?" he asked.

I was honest and direct. "I'm fucking miserable. I'm pissed and in pain. My feet are messed up, and things aren't going so great."

"Let me take a look at your feet and see if we can help."

I took a deep breath as I peeled off my shoes. I couldn't see my feet, but I did see his expression go blank as he examined them. They were an absolute mess. They had to tape them up so the blisters wouldn't fall off the bottom because that would expose raw skin. They got me wrapped up really well and after some food and a pat on the back, I was back in the wilderness with about 150 miles to go.

As I continued along the trail, I took time to rest when I needed it. One night I was settled into my sleeping bag when something woke me. I didn't just hear something; I felt the vibrations on the ground. Down the trail, I could see small glowing eyes heading toward me. The sound got increasingly louder, and I realized that it was a dogsled team heading right for me. I was sleeping on the trail and the next thing I knew, a sixteen-dog team zoomed by about a foot from my head. The musher even smiled and gave me a thumbs up.

The sheer rush of adrenaline, the power of the dogs working together, the sled slicing through the snow—it was an amazing sight to behold as humans, animals, and nature collided in a beautiful explosion. That experience gave me the motivation to continue. It was a reminder of the perseverance, the history, and the determination of everyone who puts themselves through such a brutal ordeal. I pushed myself when I woke the next morning and was soon at the 300-mile checkpoint. Only 50 miles to go! It felt like everything had finally aligned, and I'd found my stride. It had taken almost the entire route, but things had clicked, and I knew that I could finish no matter what.

Even if I was the red lantern, overcoming all those obstacles was a turning point in my life. Because I ended up in last place, I essentially ran the race against myself the entire time. I knew the others were long gone so the only real competitor, the only one who could take this victory from me, was me.

Admittedly, I'd stumbled into the event and was more enamored with the idea of competing than actually training for it. Then I'd packed a sled the size of a Prius to drag behind me for 350 miles. The odds were stacked against me. I had a slow start, I was basically laughed at, and I wasn't properly prepared. It astounded me that I was able to dig deeper than I ever had before. I was able to fall back on my athletic experience, mental strength, and sheer stubbornness and determination. When everyone doubted me, it fueled me to push through. I was able to take that negativity and turn it into a positive. I also did my share of praying and staying spiritually connected.

More importantly, I gave myself completely to the experience. Being unaware of how ill-prepared I was meant that I didn't have time to dwell on that. The jokes just fueled me to prove to myself and to everyone else that I could finish. Maybe because of my previous Alaskan adventure, I also understood the wilderness. I understood its beauty and power and mystery. That's where I felt most comfortable, and I fed off that natural energy.

Persevering and completing that race was an overwhelming combination of emotional and physical strength that had aligned perfectly. It also showed me that mentally I could overcome immense, seemingly impossible challenges if I stayed focused. When I think back to that moment, those feelings still ebb through my mind and body. I can feel my skin tingle as my mind recalls the elation.

It may not look like such an amazing accomplishment on paper. Twelve competitors finished that year, and I was No. 12. The red lantern. Last place. Runners are expected to complete the ITI in ten days. Everyone has to come in before the 11th day to be an official finisher. I completed the route in ten days with 12 hours to spare, which is kind of astounding considering all my setbacks. Still, I was a full day behind the competitor in front of me.

When I got home, I felt some embarrassment over coming in last. Granted, only 12 competitors had even finished, and I was one of them, but that didn't make me feel much better. I am a competitor at the core, so even though I realized that it was a big achievement for me, I wanted to do better.

Finishing that race against all odds garnered a lot of attention for me in the local and runner-focused press outlets. Being associated with a running store only added to my story and folks were interested in hearing about it. I was constantly asked questions about what the ITI was like and how I'd managed to keep going. It was fun to get the attention, and I enjoyed helping educate people because I didn't want anyone to jump into something like that the way I had.

I'd also recently finished running 50 marathons in 50 states, so most articles portrayed me as an intense, hyper-focused athlete who had a few stumbles along the way but never gave up. I tried my best to make sure that I didn't come across as someone with all the answers. I wanted people to understand the hardships and difficulties and how a healthy mind is as important as physical conditioning. During that time, my feet were still healing from the Alaskan punishment. It took several months to get them close to normal.

A few local groups asked me to give a talk about my experiences, and I thought it was a great idea. I was able to pull together a few photos, add in some lessons I'd learned, and provide motivational quotes that inspired me. People really seemed to respond, and the more I did it, the more expressive I became, and I learned to go deeper into stories that people enjoyed, like dragging that crazy sled through the Alaskan snow.

After each talk, I realized that something else was happening, something unexpected. Some people even commented on it. I was talking about the ITI like I planned to do it again. "Next time, I will make sure..."

In the fall of that year, I ran the Tahoe 200, and it was interesting to have other runners come up to me.

"You're the one who did the Iditarod!"

"You are one of only a dozen finishers. That's huge!"

I learned to accept and even embrace the attention. It felt good to receive their validation and accolades. I realized that the ITI is like the holy grail of ultra-events and most people will never get to experience it. So, they loved hearing the stories and couldn't get enough.

In hindsight, I would have gradually increased my physical challenges, starting with the marathons, then the 100-miler, then 200, in preparation for the ultimate 350-mile ITI. But that would be too predictable for me. I had to do it my own way, which was marathons, 100 milers, ITI, and then the Tahoe 200. Totally illogical, but somehow it worked.

Just because you can complete a certain challenge doesn't automatically mean you can crush any races that are of lesser distance. During the Tahoe 200, I reached a checkpoint and wanted to quit. I'd completed about 160 miles, and for some reason, all the cylinders were not firing. I wasn't in the zone, so I was complaining about it. During my break, I posted my concerns on Facebook, where people had started following my adventures. One guy left a comment that said, "You've got this! You've done the goddamn Iditarod. Get your ass up and get on that trail. There's no excuse not to finish." He was right, and I did finish. 202 miles in 86 hours!

In 2015, I found myself once again registered to compete in the ITI. That decision also helped my presentations because I would talk about how I was preparing for the next event and describing the things I would do differently. The next time I spoke to them, I could share my new Alaskan adventure.

I made a conscious effort to address the previous year's weaknesses. First up was the weight of the sled. During the 2014 race, I'd been afraid to run out of water, so I'd packed four huge jugs which, of course, added substantially to the weight (although they did come in handy). In 2015, I was able to pare the total weight to 45 pounds.

Then I needed to work on my navigational skills. I'd gone 25 miles off course in 2014, so I signed up for classes that included compass work and GPS hacks. Next, I needed to understand and be able to protect my feet from injury. I learned the best ways to avoid blisters, and if I did get them, when to take care of them and when to leave them alone. I was focused on being proactive this time.

It was also important to get into physical shape. I really put in the work. I worked out like a fiend and even pulled makeshift sleds around the neighborhood, where I got lots of attention and encouragement. By the time the ITI rolled around, I was in the best shape of my entire life.

At race time, Dave Johnston saw me at the hotel and said, "Goddamn, Pete, I've got to watch out for you this year!"

"I don't know about that," I said.

"You're like a different person!"

"Well, I have to be after what happened last year."

Dave picked up my sled to check the weight. This time it was genuine. He winked at me and said, "Now we're talking!"

I refer to those times when I have to dig deep inside as reaching into my pain cave. Once I hit the point of no return where I must either pull through or give up, that's when I have to get myself out of the pain cave and into the competition. I knew there would be many pain cave moments this time, but I was in great shape and hoped that would get me through any challenges. This time, it felt like I was on more equal footing with the others. I wasn't the newbie with the overweight sled.

There was also more of a camaraderie that year between me and the others. Maybe they felt I belonged. They may have just been amazed that I had the nerve to return for more after my 2014 performance. At one point, I was traveling on the trail with another guy, and it felt nice because I'd been solo the entire time the year before. I thought, *this is great, some friendly competition.* I stopped for a couple of minutes to adjust my gear and when I turned around, he was already making his way up a hill. It was a reminder that there may be some niceties, but when it came down to it, we were all on our own. There was another racer who was polite to me but a little standoffish. I got it. He had competed many times and was in a league of his own. No problem. I understand competition.

Until around the 250-mile checkpoint, I'd remained in third place for hundreds of miles. The two guys in front of me were doing their own thing. I knew there were a number of athletes behind me, but I had no idea how far back they were.

I only had about two days left before I'd reach the finish line, and I had a good stride going as I zipped across frozen lakes and waved at some of the locals. All of a sudden, a guy pulled up behind me on a snowmobile.

"Hey, you want some fireball?"

"I'm not much of a drinker. I'm good."

"How about some pot?"

That's a different story. "OK, sure, if you want to."

We stopped and he pulled out a rough-looking pipe and he started loading it with some strange weed. "Hold on, man," I told him. "I have a pipe and some of my own stuff here." At least that way I'd know what I was getting into.

We smoked and chatted back and forth for a few minutes and then he casually said, "You know, I saw another person pulling a sled just a couple miles back heading in this same direction."

I smiled, "Oh yeah? That's cool. Wait! What did you say? Someone's nearby?"

"Yeah, someone is pulling a sled just like you. He's just a few miles behind and he's heading this way."

"Holy shit, man, I gotta go!" I said as I threw my stuff back into the sled. He protested a little, but I stopped him. "I can't talk. Gotta go!"

I have never moved as fast as I did then. I was tired from a lack of sleep, but I pushed that aside and went all in. I couldn't allow complacency to be my downfall. Once I finally reached the cabin at the 350-mile finish line, one of the racers who had already finished said, "You did it, Ripmaster! You got third place," as he handed me a cold beer.

"You gotta be kidding me," I said, near tears. I couldn't believe I'd made it. I celebrated by downing the most delicious beer I'd ever had.

That year, I went into the ITI as prepared as possible and it paid off. I went from 12th place in 10½ days to third place in 6½ days. I was a machine. I was physically fit, mentally ready, and I powered through it. I had some pain cave moments, but I was happy with my performance, and it was satisfying to see how my preparation had paid off.

I was addicted and ready for a bigger challenge in 2016. Nome, like an old friend, was calling.

Chapter Eleven

Back to the Pain Cave

The stakes were much higher in 2016 because I had registered for the ITI 1,000. I'd completed the 350 twice, so I was ready for the 1,000-mile challenge. Again, I saw Dave Johnston when I arrived in Alaska, and he seemed shocked after learning of my plans.

"What the hell are you thinking?" he asked with a smile.

"You know me, Dave. I gotta try it sometime. Why not now?"

A guy named Tim was also in the race, and he was nothing short of a superstar. He had competed since 2000 and won multiple times, even setting the fastest known time in less than 20 days! He suffered for his craft and left it all on the trail. He was on a different level, and since he was competing that year, I knew he'd probably win, but I wasn't giving up or giving in.

However, my excitement for the event quickly dissipated when I noticed the landscape. Gone was the usual lush blanket of crunchy snow and glistening ice. Instead, it had been replaced with grass and rocks and dirt. It was devastating to see this beautiful terrain that thrived in the winter weather experiencing unseasonably warm conditions, no doubt a result of the global warming crisis. Not only was it a concern for the viability of the delicate ecosystem, but it meant potential issues such as rendering gear like snowshoes useless and compromised frozen lakes and streams.

The weather wasn't the only issue that year. To make matters worse, I'd fallen off short of my fitness goals at the wrong time. I'd always struggled with the strict regimen required to maintain the physique of an ultra-athlete. It's been a pattern throughout my life. Following a consistent plan indefinitely was too restrictive to me. That was my struggle in school and the traditional working world, too. Those environments thrive on policy, procedure, structure, repeatability, and predictability. All things that I am not.

So, even though I was one of only five runners invited to take on the 1,000 miles, I hadn't prepared as carefully as I should have. When I arrived, I had a noticeable gut, which may have been why Dave was so surprised. I wasn't the buff, toned Pete from 2015. However, I was confident that my persistence and general good fortune would see me through to the end. After all, that philosophy had served me well throughout my life.

As we gathered at the start line, I looked around and saw my competitors in excellent physical shape. It was obvious they had been training and honing their bodies all year in anticipation of the event. That's when I realized just how out of shape I was in comparison. It was nothing short of embarrassing, and my confidence quickly faded.

Once the race began, I knew that I didn't have the same fire in my belly. I could feel the difference. I was just going through the motions. The journey was more difficult than I'd anticipated. My body worked overtime, even on level terrain. As the trail became more treacherous, I struggled to maintain a respectable pace. All I could hear was my own labored breathing.

I stared at the deceptive beauty of the patchy winter wonderland that lay ahead. I was surrounded by huge snowbanks on either side as the white ribbon of ice and snow snaked below my feet and around the bend. After hearing the snow crackle under my feet and the harsh wind whistling through the trees for the last 200 miles, the pristine stillness felt unsettling.

I made my way around the bend, looked up at the path ahead, and felt an electric wave of fear travel through my body. The trail I was following ended abruptly and disappeared into the open water of the notoriously treacherous Tatina River. The thought of getting near exposed water made my skin tingle and sent my mind into survival mode. One slip could be fatal at those temperatures. I was in too far to retreat, so I came up with a plan.

Assessing the situation, I estimated that the water was probably waist deep at that point. I had fly fishing waders in my sled, but they would probably not be high enough. The ice water would pour right in, and I would be in an even more dangerous situation. There was no denying that it would be life-threatening for me to try crossing there. My only other option was to travel either far left or far right of the main trail.

Right looked like certain death to me. I looked to the left and saw a set of footprints along the ice that I assumed meant someone had successfully crossed the river and most likely linked back up to the main trail. *OK*, I thought, *so this won't be so bad. Someone has already been here so it must be possible.* All I needed to do was follow those steps, and I'd be back on the solid ground of the main trail. I felt a sense of relief as I began to methodically work my way across the river using my trekking poles to test the ice. If I found a weak spot, I could adjust my path to avoid that area. It would be painstaking and tedious, but at least I'd be safe. It wasn't about coming in first place at this point. It was about survival.

So, I began tapping the poles on the ice ahead of me. Then I'd slide my feet along and repeat the pattern. Tink, Tink. Swoosh, Swoosh. Getting into a rhythm helped me push the fear aside and focus on the task ahead of me. After keeping up a steady pace, I finally looked up and thought, *I'm halfway across the damn river!* I could feel my heartbeat slow down and my blood pressure subside. With my confidence restored, it was just a matter of time before I'd be off this dangerous section and back on track.

I smiled as I extended the poles and drove them into the ice ahead. Tink, Tink. Swoosh, Swoosh. Then I did it again, but this time I heard a loud pop, and a fracture line zipped right under my feet. I was momentarily weightless as the ice gave way beneath me. Instinctively, I took in a gasp of air before the freezing water swallowed me whole. My body was tossed left and right by the rushing current. I fought to reach the surface, but the icy water gripped me like a vise, pulling me back down. I knew I only had a few seconds before I'd need more air, so I stabbed my arms toward the surface, finally pulling myself upward. When I reached the top, I gasped for precious air as I dog-paddled to stay afloat. I felt a tug below me and remembered my sled was still attached, swirling in the dark water below.

Each time I tried to pull myself up on the ice, it would break off. I was treading water and desperately trying to figure out how to reach the other side of the river. I had no concept of time, so I don't know how long it took, but I finally found enough purchase on an ice bank to roll my body out of the water. I lay there, assessing the mess I'd gotten myself into. Mistakes can be deadly in this unforgiving terrain. I was out of the water but soaking wet in the dark, bone-chilling night. Not only that, I still had to travel three or four miles on the river before getting to the next checkpoint.

I felt myself hyperventilating, so I tried to focus on slowing down my breathing. I thought about my wife, my daughters, my life, and I just lay there crying and cursing my situation. Throughout all my adventures, there was always an element of danger, but I'd never found myself in such dire straits. I was glad I'd been able to pull myself out of the water, but then I realized, fuck, my sled, which was still attached, was still under water with all my gear. Somehow, I found the strength to pull slowly and carefully until I was able to bring my sled to the surface. It was heavily covered with ice, and I realized that I was, too. My clothing was brittle, and everything was hopelessly saturated.

Plus, I was still in the middle of the river. There were no trees or brush, so if I needed to make a fire, I still had to go hundreds of yards to reach the bank. Then maybe I could dump my fuel over a tree and throw a spark so that there'd be enough warmth to dry off some of my gear before getting back on the trail. My other option was to keep moving toward the next checkpoint, which was a few miles away. I wasn't sure if I had the strength, but I decided to give it a shot. I was in a messed up mental state—crying, shaking, scared as hell that I wasn't going to make it. Then I heard something familiar.

Widespread Panic was blasting from my headphones. I had been listening to them while I was hiking. I still loved that band, and I'd had that awkward first date with my wife at one of their concerts. For some reason, remembering that helped ground me and gave me the motivation to get up and begin moving. Several times I wiped my eyes so that I could scan the pure white landscape for a glimpse of the checkpoint. Every step was calculated and steady, and I was elated when I was finally able to make out a clearing in the woods up ahead.

The volunteers from the more famous sled dog race had a heated cabin at the wilderness checkpoint of Rohn. ITI racers were provided with more rustic accommodations and were discouraged from entering the nicer cabin. I opened the door of the ITI wall tent and peeked inside. There was no one; not even a fire going. It was as cold inside as out. I saw a plume of smoke wafting from the other cabin, made my way over, and knocked on the door. Before they could turn me away, I pushed inside and blurted out that I had fallen into the river.

Several volunteers were staying at the cabin while preparing the area for the mushers and dogs that would arrive in a few days. A couple of guys helped me strip out of my clothes and got me near the fire to warm up and dry off my gear while the women tried to give me privacy in the tight quarters. I was experiencing a rush of emotions because I was so happy to be alive, but that narrow escape really messed with my mind, and I began laughing uncontrollably. Someone pulled out a giant bottle of whiskey, and we took a few refreshing, belly-warming shots. I was going to be ok.

Once my gear was dry, I had to take stock. Do I keep going? I'd already completed 200 miles. I had 800 to go before reaching Nome. It was a difficult decision because once I set my mind to something, it's as good as done. Despite the death-defying river escape, I still felt that I could make it with my dried-out gear and a recharged spirit of adventure. I also knew that my family, friends, and others in my town were following my journey on a website using a GPS tracker. There was a lot of support behind me, and I couldn't fathom letting everyone down. Since I wasn't carrying a satellite phone during this race, someone gave me one to use.

As soon as I heard the sweet, familiar voice of home, I said, "Kristen, I fell in the river! The ice gave way! I went fully underwater! I thought it was over!"

"Pete, I know. Where are you now? How are you feeling?"

"At the checkpoint. I'm OK. Dry, recharged, I'm good."

"Are you flying home?" she asked.

"No, I'm gonna finish it. I have to."

"I know," she said quietly.

I began calculating the mileage in my head. It's something I did on the trail to keep my mind active and out of dark places. I'd already covered 200 miles. There were 300 more to the 500-mile mark. Halfway. I felt confident that I could do it. So, I packed up and hit the trail once again. I continued hiking at a speed of almost three miles an hour, averaging about 37 miles a day, until I was just outside the town of Ruby which I knew sat on the Yukon River. On the northern route that I was taking, the Yukon marked the halfway point of the race. Convinced that I could do it, I made a 15-mile uphill climb to the top of a mountain with views of Ruby.

I looked out at the rugged terrain that surrounded me, and I remembered to soak in the moment. It was hard to believe that I was almost swallowed by the Tatina, but I'd not only survived; I'd also persevered. My prayers had been answered, and my faith had seen me through. Going 500 more miles would be brutal, but up on that mountain it felt possible. Then I looked down. Miles below, the mighty Yukon lay still, but I knew better. There was no way in hell I was going anywhere near it. To be honest, it scared the shit out of me and looked like an ocean instead of a river. Those first 200 miles almost took my life and I'd still managed to go another 300, but I was not going to tempt fate a second time by stepping foot on that river. Sometimes, the smartest survival technique is knowing when to call it quits.

I could see that Ruby was only about three miles away. That sealed the deal for me. I'd check in there and tap out. Done. Finished. See you later, Alaska! I still had to get down the hill, so I looked back at my sled and thought, *Since I'm quitting, I am going to ride this thing!* I'd wanted to do that many times, but it was a risky move. Now, what did I have to lose? Why not go out in style? I hopped on the sled and held my poles behind me to make sure I could maneuver around anything in the way. With a mighty shove, I was quickly sailing down the snowy hill at about 20 miles an hour, taking the bumps, catching air a few times, my goggles on and a goofy smile plastered on my face. I felt like a kid out of school on a snow day. I passed two native Alaskans working on a truck in their driveway. They looked at me like I was insane. I think they understood something I hadn't even thought about: I'd need to stop at some point.

Just then, a snowbank appeared out of nowhere, and I crashed into it face first and flopped over on my back, the sled askew under a pile of snow. I laughed as I dusted myself off and waved at the guys to let them know I was OK. Then I trekked over to the checkpoint where one of the other ITI racers was unpacking his gear.

"Hey, you made it," Eric Johnson said. "Sweet, man! I'm so glad. I'm going to take a 24-hour rest here. Why don't you do the same? Then we'll regroup and head out together."

I looked at him and shook my head. "No, I'm done."

"No, man, you can't. You're halfway, dude. You're golden! Come on!"

"I'm done. That's it."

Soon I was on a plane going from Ruby to Fairbanks, then to Anchorage. The thing is, I forgot to take off my tracker so the people back home who were watching my progress saw my dot on the map zooming along at about 500 miles an hour! That's how they knew something was up.

That night, I was sitting in a hotel room in Anchorage, eating pizza, and watching SportsCenter when I began to question myself. *What did I just do? I was halfway through! Why did I stop? Yeah, I cheated death, but that's part of the adventure.* Remarkably, there wasn't anything physically wrong with me. For a split second, I considered getting back on the plane and having them drop me off where I'd stopped racing so I could just keep going. Then I had to reason with myself. "Nope, you knew what you were doing. You stopped for a reason, and you're gonna make a big boy decision here and fly home. Quit second-guessing yourself."

Not finishing was one of the hardest things I'd ever done. For me, it was much harder than the actual race. But I understood that it was something I had to do. I needed to celebrate and honor the fact that I was alive. No matter who I told the story to, no one would really understand what it was like to feel how fragile life can be out there in the wilderness. I needed to reconnect with my family. I was able to make peace with that decision because of all the self-work I'd already done. I'd fought hard to manage the demons and conquer the darkness that consumed much of my life, and I didn't want to backslide now.

On the way home, I made a deal with myself. I'd accept this defeat like a man and be clear with everyone about how it was the best choice for me at that moment. If they didn't understand, that was their problem. This was my journey and mine alone.

In retrospect, that year was the combination of an untoned body, a flawed training regimen, and the warm temperatures that blanketed Alaska. There were too many strikes against me from the jump. My stubborn streak and Ripmaster luck were no match for the mighty Tatina. The ice never had a chance to fully form, and I quickly found myself pulled under as sub-zero waters yanked my body left and right like a chubby ragdoll. For a split second, as I thrashed under the freezing water, I felt I was going to die.

The race had been miserable, and I allowed self-doubt to creep in. The nagging depression that I usually kept at bay was circling my brain as tightly as the water gipping my body. It would have been so easy to surrender to the powerful river. Who would blame me? I would have gotten exactly what I deserved. As an experienced athlete at this stage in my career,

I knew better than to arrive half-cocked at one of the world's most challenging physical tests. Yet, I had done exactly that.

The strength I had to summon to get myself out of that situation came from deep down in the depths of my soul. I pushed away the evil thoughts that depression dangled in front of me and dug deep. I did it for my daughters. I did it for Kristen. And I did it to prove to myself that the dark thoughts would not win. They would not dictate my fate, no matter how dire the circumstances. My stubborn ass wouldn't allow it.

Despite everything working against me, I saved my skin and reached the halfway point before calling it quits. I did not see it as quitting. To me, that means giving up when you still have more to give. In that situation, I knew that it was time to stop. That harrowing Yukon River had told me loud and clear that it was time to cut bait.

The worst part of the entire experience was not even what happened on the trail. News of a runner who got swallowed up by the Tatina River spread quickly because people watch the yearly event from all over the world. I later found out that Kristen was reading a *USA Today* article about an athlete who nearly died on the Iditarod, and as she kept reading, she realized the article was about me. I had not been able to contact her directly at that point. It cut me to the core to think about how she must have felt reading about her own husband.

As soon as I was able, I called to let her know that I had quit and was coming home early. That is when she told me about the article she'd read. This time, my lack of preparation had almost cost me my life and had scared my family. I could not let that ever happen again, so I quickly assured Kristen that I wouldn't attempt the ITI again. It was too risky.

She was quiet for a second before she said, "Pete, we both know you can't say that. It makes sense that you had to stop early, but you would never forgive yourself if you didn't go back next year."

Naturally, she was right. I had said that because I thought that was what she wanted and needed to hear. And I meant it. If she didn't want me to do it again, to avoid putting her through more worry, I wouldn't. However, she added that we both knew it would haunt me if I didn't try again. Yeah, I made the decision to quit, but that didn't mean I was giving up. In fact, I was just getting started.

Undeterred, I signed up for the 2017 race. I was either a glutton for punishment or more determined than Sisyphus pushing that boulder up a mountain. Every time I thought I'd made headway reaching my goal, I found myself back at square one. I had been dreaming of the Iditarod since childhood. The dogsled version wasn't right for me, but the ITI was perfect. It was incredibly frustrating because I knew inside that I could do it. I could visualize finishing the 1,000, but I hadn't been able to make it happen.

The 2017 race marked my fourth ITI and my second attempt at 1,000 miles on foot. My fixation on finishing was not only affecting me but was also taking a toll on my entire family. I was more apprehensive because of what had happened the last year. Facing that damn river again would be tough. Honestly, I wasn't sure if I could do it. Plus, I knew everyone in my family was concerned about the dangers that I would face. Hunter was born in 2008 and Reagan in 2011, so both girls were now old enough to be aware of the challenges and dangers of my adventures. It came to the point where I'd leave the house after the kids went to bed to avoid the inevitable tears.

That year, the typical Alaskan winter was back in all its glory. The glistening snow engulfed the landscape with its undeniable allure. The temperature hovered around minus-20 degrees Fahrenheit with the northern winds factored in. For me, it was a welcome cold. I knew it would add more difficulty in many ways, but I embraced it as a sign of good fortune and frozen rivers.

Everything was copacetic in that race for the first 150 miles or so. It was challenging but not particularly eventful, which is exactly what a racer wants. No surprises are a good thing. Slow and steady and focused, that was my mantra. I was not going to let that river or anything else intimidate me or shake my determination. I had gone about 165 miles in four days when I reached the last checkpoint before entering the dense wilderness. It was the Rainy Pass Lodge, and it would be the last checkpoint for about 40 miles or so.

Right away, I noticed something alarming. Those checkpoints were usually deserted, with maybe one racer taking a break. This time, the cabin was packed with folks who had turned around and come back because of the unusually harsh weather. The wind had kicked up, ushering in an intense cold that most could not withstand. They had realized that if they went too far, it would be much more difficult to return to the checkpoint and they could be stranded.

I still had more than 800 miles to go, so I took a brief rest and then prepared to leave. I didn't want their reluctance to inform my decision. Just because they weren't comfortable continuing didn't necessarily mean I couldn't.

With my goggles snug and several layers covering my face, I soldiered on. The punishing winds became so intense that I was often forced to walk backward as the snow continued to pelt me with every step. After about 20 miles of the unrelenting weather, I understood just how formidable it was and why most folks had decided to turn back.

I happened upon one racer burrowed down in his sleeping bag with snow piling up around him. I screamed as loud as I could to be heard over the howling wind, but there was no movement. I reached him and began pushing on him. "Hey, are you OK? It's Pete."

He lifted his head slowly and hollered over the wind. "I could hear your sled dragging along the ice from miles away. I just had to stop. Man, I can't handle this weather."

"Well, then I'm going to stop, too," I yelled. "I'm not going to leave you here alone! We can stick together!"

He nodded and I settled in nearby, careful not to remove my shoes, because if they froze, I wouldn't be able to get them back on. That next hour was probably even more harrowing than falling through the ice. The temperature continued to fall, and the wind was brutal. There was no escaping it. I lay inside my sleeping bag, fully covered in layers. Then I could feel my muscles tightening and loosening quickly in an effort to warm up. I was shivering harder than ever before, and I couldn't stop it.

It had taken about 30 minutes to get settled, but it was obvious that I couldn't stay there in -60F temperatures. If I fell asleep, I might never wake up. The lull of slumber, the ability to temporarily escape the cold was alluring, but the result could be deadly. I had to keep moving.

"I can't sleep in this weather," I yelled. "I have to keep moving. Come on!"

He shook his head and bellowed, "No, I'm tired. I'm staying here until the sun comes up. Go ahead!"

Because I couldn't keep warm, I had no choice. So, I continued down the trail, pushing through the swirling snow and stinging wind until I was stopped in my tracks, unable to go on. A wave of fear pulsed through my body as the snow danced around me. There it was, the Tatina River. I knew that eventually the moment would come, yet the weather and treacherous conditions had kept my mind occupied. Now there was no escaping the fact that I'd have to cross that river again.

It is difficult to explain the feeling of being in such horrendous weather with no one around for miles and miles. It must be the way explorers felt when traveling new territories with no idea of what they would encounter. It was scary to realize that life or death was completely dependent upon my next move. There was no one to call if I needed help.

To reach the next checkpoint, I had to settle the score with the Tatina. Kristen was tracking me, so I knew she had been bracing for that moment. This time, I was careful to assess the situation although it was much more difficult because of the weather. One of the consequences of falling through the ice was that I remembered every detail clearly. It was etched into my memory, so I harnessed that knowledge as I approached.

Carefully. Slowly. Cautiously. I slowed down and focused to avoid any distractions. I pushed back the natural instinct to turn around, the urge to protect myself from the danger lurking below the surface. The punishing weather was a benefit in that situation because the ice was surely frozen. As long as I avoided any compromised areas where logs or branches had fallen through and broken the surface, I should be safe. I distracted my mind with the small tasks at hand as I slid my feet, one at a time, carefully pulling my sled, stopping to dislodge it when necessary. If I looked too far ahead, the memories would return, so I stayed present and gradually made my way across.

When I reached the other side, I felt my muscles unclench and my body relax for a moment. I was so relieved that I'd not only conquered the river, but, more importantly, I hadn't allowed the accident to define my performance. Once safely across, I tried my phone signal and was able to call home. It felt amazing to share that victory with Kristen and reassure her that I had made it.

The checkpoint at McGrath was about 350 miles into the 1,000-mile race. Of the approximately 40 athletes, only four of us made it that far. The others racing on foot had decided not to continue because of the weather. Within our quartet, two had planned to stop at the 350, and two of us were going all the way to the end.

The other 1,000-mile racer turned to me and said, "There's no way I'm attempting the journey to Nome."

I had two choices. One was to travel 650 miles by myself with little likelihood of seeing anyone else; the other was to stop at the 350 and call it a day. After conquering not only that river but my internal doubts as well, I was dripping in ego and could picture the headlines "Ripmaster! The Only ITI Racer to Tough It Out!" It was one of those defining moments for an endurance athlete that can make or break a career in competitive racing. Was this an opportunity I would regret if I didn't take it? Should I be the lone wolf and push through despite the bad weather? Should I risk my safety again?

I could see there was real career potential and lifetime bragging rights; however, I knew for a fact that it was not smart to go it alone in that weather. It was potentially suicidal to make the decision based on ego. That's when I decided that after analyzing the situation, as any survivalist should, I would stop at the 350. It was a conscious decision not to question or second-guess myself, which I had a tendency to do.

It was more difficult because I had already crossed the river, I'd made smart choices throughout the race, and the only issue was the brutal weather. It was somewhat of a concession that I'd completed the 350 and consciously opted out of the 1,000, so it didn't look like a failure to others; but if I'm honest, it did feel like one to me.

I had been giving talks in and around Asheville for a while, and after I returned from the 2017 race, I had an appearance where only eight people showed up. It really hit me hard because I already felt defeated by the race and then it looked like no one cared that I had finished the 350 once again. Everyone was counting on me to at least attempt the 1,000. When I heard that a few racers on bicycles had gone all the way to Nome after discovering clear weather just past the 350-mile mark, it hurt. It hurt a lot.

That familiar push and pull began to dance inside my head, that feeling that I usually fail to recognize until it has a firm hold on my soul. I have tried all my life to "manage" my depression. I am just not sure it's possible. No matter how hard I worked to identify it, compartmentalize it, and deal with it, I always seemed to end up in the same smothering spiral of despair and dread. It was frustrating as hell, and I just wanted the ability to focus without the noise.

It felt strange to be home earlier than expected because that was a clear sign to everyone that I had not hit my goal. Since it was such big news around town, it felt like everyone was judging me behind their smiles and nods. It is natural to welcome a winner home, but what about when you're not a winner? I can tell you the welcome is much less enthusiastic. That's for sure.

Kristen and the girls had made plans to spend time with family while I was away, and since I was back early, it felt like I was crashing the party at my own house. Smiling and answering questions was pure torture because I just didn't feel good about it, no matter how much I tried to convince myself otherwise.

To cope, I decided to go camping by myself for a couple of days to clear my head and make peace with everything, starting with myself. What if I can never do it? Who am I? Who do I want to be? Have I overestimated my abilities? Will I be able to live with that truth?

I had to decide if I wanted to try yet again in 2018. If I did that, I'd have to think about my performance every day and night for a full year. Back when I played baseball, my coach told me I was one of the best two-strike hitters he had ever seen. I never got nervous when there were two strikes against me; I always came through under pressure.

Good athletes know their limits, and maybe I'd reached mine. There was one way to find out. I decided to make 2018 my final attempt at the ITI 1,000.

Chapter Twelve

Nome Sweet Nome

When I was living in Colorado, I adopted Percy, a wolf hybrid who was only a few weeks old and the size of a six-pack of beer. He had intense eyes and grew to be fiercely loyal. I took that pup everywhere, and we explored hundreds of miles of trails together. At 15 years old, he weighed about 110 pounds and began having trouble navigating the stairs at our house. It was two weeks before the 2018 ITI, and I made the heart-wrenching decision to relieve him of his pain even though it would, in turn, magnify mine.

Any pet lover knows how horrible that moment is, no matter how much we rationalize it. Even though it's for the best, that doesn't make it any less painful. He and I had been together before I started a family, and he was my trusty sidekick. I could count on him to be up for any adventure, and he kept me sane when I felt out of control.

Losing Percy was a sharp reminder that I'd lost many of those I loved, including of course Mom and then Dad. My first instinct was to retreat into myself, to self-reflect, and to take stock of my life, but I didn't have that luxury. The ITI was fast approaching, and I needed to stay focused.

In past years, I had been supported by a running company that acted as an informal sponsor. As with previous events, I emailed them about the upcoming race. *Hey, I'm getting ready to try the ITI one more time. I could use a few pairs of those shoes that I usually get. Can you send them in time?* My contact at the company wrote back and said sure, just let them know what I needed. It felt good to have them on my side, and then I decided to scroll down.

He had accidentally forwarded the entire email trail that had been sent around the company. I read past a message that said, *Sure, we're here for you, Pete. Go get 'em.* The next one said, *Pete's going back out to Alaska again.* Another read, *He probably won't finish, just like the other years.* And another, *We won't use any of this on our social media unless we get desperate.* The more I read, the more pissed off I got. How could they not understand that was how competition worked? No one goes in and wins everything right away. It takes time. It takes perseverance. It takes decent shoes!

It upset me so much because that negativity only served to feed my ever-present doubts and misgivings about returning to the ITI. Was I being stubborn? Was I overestimating my abilities? Could everyone see something that I was missing? They seemed to have no concept of what it took to almost lose your life in that river and keep going back. Didn't they understand only a dozen people had ever even finished the 1,000 in 18 years? To top it off, I had just lost my buddy Percy, so I was in a vulnerable place anyway.

I hastily pounded out an email to shoot back to them saying, *Thanks but no thanks. How dare you treat me with such disrespect!* That was one of those moments where mindfulness and personal peace came into play. I realized that maybe there was some truth to what they were saying. That might be how people were feeling about me. They would never understand why that event was one of the toughest on the planet. They just wanted a winner, like everyone else. So, I took the mature route and deleted the email. Then, I centered myself, compartmentalized my frustrations, and made a conscious effort to channel those feelings into my performance at the race. I would use that negativity to fuel my determination.

Through my previous races, I'd learned a lot about how to navigate the ITI and the Alaskan wilderness. From packing to camping to interactions with locals, thoughtful choices were critical. One wrong move could spell defeat.

When it came to packing my bag, my choices were much more calculated than my initial attempt in 2014. I had five years of experience learning what worked and, more importantly, what didn't. One of the important lessons was finding multiple uses for anything I packed because space on that sled was precious, and each ounce of weight would impact my performance.

Typically, a smartly packed sled rounds out at about 45 pounds fully loaded. There were no hard and fast rules on what could or couldn't be packed. Most athletes had their own strategy. It was really up to individual preference, and I found that their packing style was a good barometer of their personality. Some athletes were a bit standoffish, preferring to stay in a competitive headspace. Their packs were often minimal, taking just the absolute necessities. Then there were the gear heads wearing headphones and stocking up on the latest high-tech gadgets designed to make the journey more efficient, or at least more bearable. Some of the international athletes insisted on creature comforts like food preparation gear and padded bedding. The newbies usually threw in everything but the kitchen sink, something I was guilty of on my first attempt. Typically, the more experienced a racer was, the more streamlined their pack.

I would never again attempt to pull a sled that tipped the scales at almost 100 pounds as I did in 2014. I used my on-the-trail experiences to make better packing decisions. It was not about tossing in survival gear until I reached the target weight. My approach was to carefully consider each item, its weight, and its usability. I couldn't afford any extra pounds this time. A hastily packed sled could derail everything...again.

To make the cut, anything I packed had to be essential for either clothing, food/water, shelter, or navigation. If not, then it had to go. That meant I even avoided packing reminders of home, despite the urge to include them. After my past mistakes, I was now focused on traveling as light as possible. It was a personal challenge that I'd issued to myself.

That strategy paid off, and my sled was noticeably lighter than previous years. Returning racers who remembered my packing challenges came up and commented, "Is that all you're bringing this time?" Funny. In the past, those comments would have caused me to get into my head, but not this time. My focus was strong, my conviction was firm, and my pack was on point.

As far as clothing, extra socks were non-negotiable. They were a must. If they got wet, it was almost impossible to dry them out in those frigid temperatures. Stepping in a mound of snow or breaking through fragile ice could easily allow moisture to slip in no matter how high your boots were. I took just one pair of shoes and boots that I could slip over my socks. That was a gamble because if something happened to those shoes, it could be a derailer; but I was willing to risk it. If my shoes happened to blow out, my plan was to just double up on the socks and wear my overboots since they were made to withstand 40-below temperatures. As it turned out, I only needed my boots on occasion. Otherwise, my shoes gave me more mobility and speed on the trails.

I did pack extra clothes to have on hand because layering was crucial. However, you can only wear a finite number of clothes, so it was important for me to exercise restraint. For me, when I'm out on the trail, even if it's freezing out, I work up a sweat. I don't know what it's like for others but pulling a 50-pound sled through the snow is an intense workout and I warm up fast. Too many layers can inhibit my performance and make me uncomfortable.

To cope with that, I played a little game where I tried to get by with as few layers as possible while still keeping warm, without sacrificing performance. The trick comes when I have to stop for any reason. Whether it's to take a pee break, have a snack, or get my bearings, once I'm still for a minute or so, the cold creeps in and I am back to square one. Time to layer up again. It's a repeatable cycle that I try to manage as efficiently as possible throughout the race.

One article of clothing that I could not go without was my "bombproof coat." It was made of heavy Gore-Tex with an arctic fur lining, and I considered it a dear friend. It was my go-to when that Alaskan wind sliced down off the mountain and practically blew me off the trail. My bomber coat was designed to sustain 60-below temperatures. When there wasn't a checkpoint for another 30 miles and the sun was hiding behind a silver band of clouds, that coat was a lifesaver.

One of my least favorite things to do on the trail was to stop and retrieve something from the sled. For me, it was a domino effect in which I'd get something and that would lead to something else that I thought I needed. It's all about time management. If I had to stop, remove the harness that I wear to pull the sled, untie my pack and open it up, that was precious trail time that I'd spent so it had better be worth it. It was easy for me to fall into the trap of thinking that since the pack was open, I might as well pull out other things while I was there. Maybe I should reorganize the food and count how many dry socks I had. And I could always use a water refill. Before I realized it, that quick stop clocked in at an hour and a half of me fussing with my pack.

I had to remember that my strategy was to try my hardest to avoid stopping until I'd reached my next destination. Very often that meant I was a wreck once I got there. I'd have sweat seeping through my layers, and I'd be smelly, hungry, and tired. Not all athletes function like that, but by 2018, that method was working for me. Once I reached a shelter, I would take time to regroup, re-pack if necessary, and clean up. I preferred eating and sleeping there instead of on the trail if I could help it. Being out of the elements allowed me to reset and get my head back in the game.

Some of the athletes took a completely different approach and were perfectly content to stop every few hours for a break or maybe a quick meal. That's one reason I was never able to travel using the buddy system because I found it tough to compromise when I felt it was detracting from my performance. I liked to keep moving. Stillness was the enemy.

When I did sleep on the trail, I had my bivy, which was a thin, lightweight outer bag that went around my sleeping bag and floor mat. It was like a little tent that kept the elements out as much as possible. I also took along a very basic medical kit, but nothing extensive.

That year, one of my packing splurges was to bring electronics, but I was judicious in my approach because they often turned out to be more of a hinderance. If they weren't used often, they took up precious space. Also, some electronics were ineffective in extreme temperatures and the cords were frustrating, so that was a consideration.

I found that out because I was adamant about taking my iPod. Being on the trails for days on end, it can get tedious and lonely. Having music for inspiration and motivation can help but keeping it charged and managing the tangled cords and plugs was a distraction for me. I also took my GPS, and a satellite phone because cell service was a rarity in the Alaskan wilderness.

For those times when I did have to stop on the trail, I had packed a stove, a pot, and a few meals. Truth be told, I probably could have gone without those things except they were handy when it was necessary to melt snow for water. Otherwise, I didn't have the patience to prepare a meal. I'd rather eat prepackaged food and keep it moving, although that strategy definitely took a toll on my health.

Going back to Alaska was my chance to either hit a home run or strikeout and concede defeat. There was no in-between. No middle ground. I hated the two days before the race because all the athletes were gathered around talking about their gear and the races they had won and their future plans. It just drove me crazy because my only focus was the ITI, not impressing anyone else. The photo of me at the 2014 race was that of a grinning idiot, a complete rookie. At the start of the 2018 ITI, it was the polar opposite. I looked like I was possessed. I was intense and focused, like a caged greyhound just waiting to be let loose.

The race started promptly at 2:00 p.m. Once that .44 was shot into the air, the riders on their fat-tired bikes went first and that meant everyone on foot or skis was in the back. I took the opportunity to make my way up front among the bikers. I didn't care if they liked it or not, I had as much right to be there as they did. Most participants were planning to stop at 350 miles, so even though they were not my competition, it felt like a boss move.

The bikers would be done before those on foot unless they ran into a mechanical issue. So, it wouldn't do me any good to get too caught up in the race at the beginning, but I wanted to make sure everyone knew I was serious. Previously, I would go straight through the night to reach the aid station at mile 59 at 6:00 in the morning. Then, after just a couple of hours of sleep, I'd keep going until the next checkpoint. It was a brutal pace and possibly my downfall.

That year, I promised myself that if I felt good about my performance, I would stop the first night at about 30 miles in, right by one of the big rivers. However, it was tough to follow through on that because the others kept passing me by, and as a competitor, I couldn't train myself to remain still as they continued on. Fortunately, I was able to reach down deep and stay the course. I was determined to follow a different plan that time. To my surprise, I actually got a good night's sleep. It was freezing cold, but I woke up refreshed and ready to go.

It felt good to know that I was not allowing anyone else's decisions to impact my performance. Sticking to the plan *was* the plan. No deviations. No second-guesses. I kept thinking; *this is your year. It's all coming together.* That didn't mean much when I had over 800 miles to go, but it helped, and it gave me something to hold on to even after I'd made a huge mistake.

After leaving a checkpoint at about 135 miles into the race, I traveled another 40 miles or so before it got super cold. I allowed myself to stop moving and go into my sled for the old reliable bomber coat. Once I started fishing around, I came to the crushing realization that I had left it at the last checkpoint. It was a devastating blow because no matter how much I had planned and strategized, one mistake could mean the end of my race.

I started to beat myself up for being so careless. It was an easy mistake to make, but I knew better. That was one of the times when my reluctance to stop was a liability. Had I taken a break maybe ten miles out from the pit stop just to double-check everything, I could have easily headed back even though that would have added 20 unnecessary miles to my race. However, being 40 miles away meant 80 additional miles if I turned back.

On the other hand, it was so early in the race, relatively speaking, that I would have to get through almost 900 miles without my warmest coat. Because of that, I did contemplate going back to retrieve it. Frequently, if that happens and someone finds something important that has been left behind, they will find someone who could deliver it to the next checkpoint. But there was no guarantee that would happen. Even if it did, the timing could be off, and I may have needed to wait there for a delivery that might never arrive. It was yet another one of those times when I had to rely on my instincts to make the choice that was right for me in that moment. I decided to press on.

If I were serious about this race, I couldn't allow one mistake to turn into two. Leaving the coat was already a done deal. I had to layer up, press on, and hope for the best. Naturally, when I arrived at the next checkpoint, I asked about my coat with hope in my heart. Yet, they had no idea what I was talking about. Just my luck. It was my error, and I made peace with that as I continued. There was no denying that it was brutal, especially anytime I stopped along the trail with the cold seeping into my bones.

As I trudged along the winding, snow-covered trails, the checkpoints were a mixed bag. There were about 50 miles or so between each shelter and the accommodations varied wildly. Along the 1,000 miles, maybe a dozen were nice, comfortable rest stops. Others were little more than a decrepit cabin that had been neglected for years.

It was important for me to manage my expectations because there was no consistency among the stops. It was great to be out of the elements, but the conditions inside varied widely. For the most part, I could deal with the chaos as long as I could get some sleep without having to lay on the hard, bitter cold snow.

At one stop, I was so exhausted my only thought was to pass out, but the distractions were intense. There were ten other athletes squeezed inside and some were coughing and throwing up, others were complaining about the trail. A couple were huddled on the floor snoring loudly. One guy was on the phone actually crying to his wife about something, while another tended to his blistered feet near the pot of stew. It truly was mayhem.

That year, I was beyond focused and found the chaos not only irritating, but it distracted me from my mission. I purposely avoiding being sucked into anyone's issues or drama because I needed to keep my eye on the prize. All I wanted to do was check my gear, charge my equipment, and possibly sleep a little before moving on.

As a result, during that race, I'd reach a checkpoint and quickly poke my head in the door. If there was too much going on, I'd keep going and sleep along the trail if I had to. Because I was pushing myself so hard, sleep was important to me. It sometimes made more sense to crash on the trail and avoid the checkpoint mayhem.

There were a couple of really nice stops along the way. They even allowed racers to pre-order meals and rent a private room for the right price. That was true luxury after traveling for days on end in the brutal weather. Some had heaters, a bed off the floor, and a shower. I would walk out of one of those checkpoints feeling like a new person. Having that uninterrupted time to take care of any health issues like chafing or blisters, sleeping a full six or seven hours, and feeling clean had a way of improving even the worst mood. It was the mental reset that I needed; however, those places were few and far between. Most were primitive at best.

At one point in the race, I'd been hiking for 70 miles or so, staying up two nights in a row, with hardly any food. After trudging for a few more hours through a snowstorm, I struggled to reach the shelter cabin up ahead that was marked as the next checkpoint. Upon my arrival, there were 15 high-end snow machines parked around the perimeter and the front door was locked. These guys were locals or tourists who rode snowmobiles and followed the Iditarod dog sled racers along the trail. Then they would take over an entire cabin, which could mean life or death for the ITI racers.

I pulled on the front door, but it wouldn't budge. I knew that without a dog sled, other racers were seen as inconsequential to them. Their focus was on the celebrated dog racers, and they didn't care about those on foot, bikes, or skis. That happened more than I expected. There were a few times when I'd hike for days, struggling to make it to a checkpoint where I could get a meal and, because it was late at night, they would not be as welcoming as I'd hoped. It wasn't that I needed a party or anything, just basic comfort and a chance to rest. Some of the checkpoints were even located in the houses of locals who would rent out rooms. They weren't always excited to see hungry, smelly racers in the middle of the night while their kids slept in the next room.

At a couple of checkpoints, I tried to use earplugs, but that didn't work for me. I couldn't shut out the noise no matter how hard I tried. It was emotionally taxing to travel so far without having any idea what type of reception would be waiting on the other side of the door.

The one near mile 59 was a family home where they had a few rooms that were available on a first-come basis. I had to remind myself to be respectful and gracious even though I was so exhausted that I could barely stand up. The next one was more like an Alaskan lodge that even had a restaurant where racers could order a meal. Another was little more than a hunting cabin; that was the one I had struggled to reach after I fell into the Tatina. It was incredibly primitive.

Nikolai was the first town I reached along the trail. The Nikolai village was a federally recognized tribe, and they made up the majority of the population. It was a stopover during the Gold Rush with a trading post and roadhouse, and now a checkpoint for the Iditarod. They had a rec hall where racers could eat, spread out, and re-energize. It was nice to get out of the weather for a bit and catch my breath.

Back on the trail, I felt rundown and as tired as a worn-out shoe. I was between checkpoints and realized my only option was to sleep outside, and that was fine. I was prepared for it. After about 45 minutes of setup, I was ready to huddle up by the trail and get some shut eye.

I'd just acclimated to the unforgiving snow and drifted off when the next thing I knew, I was grazed by a snowmobile that sped by only inches from my head. It had to be traveling around 70 mph. Before I could even collect my thoughts, I saw the headlights swing around and bounce along the snow before they headed back in my direction!

That was a close call, and I was in no mood for their games. I hopped out of my sleeping bag and steeled myself for a confrontation. Like I always say, it was not the animals I worried about as much as the thrill seekers looking for trouble. Once the snowmobile got closer, it slowed down and pulled up beside me. There were two guys, and I could smell the alcohol right away. One of them tried to speak, but I couldn't understand him because he was slurring his words. They were completely bombed, and for some reason they were angry.

I couldn't figure out what the actual problem was, but the skinny one in the front was gesturing wildly. The man in the back had to be around 400 pounds or so and he was even worse off. Another reason the entire situation was odd was because there were rarely two people on one ride.

Then the larger one said, "Where's McGrath?"

It was an unusual question because the locals were asking me, an obvious outsider, for directions. I had already planned my route for the next day, so I knew exactly how to get there. I pointed in the direction and said, "It's that way." They began to argue with me that I was wrong and didn't know what I was talking about. I had learned from experience there was no reasoning with someone that messed up, so I just said, "Ok, well, believe what you want. You asked me a question, and I answered you. I was trying to sleep when you guys buzzed right by my head."

That got them more agitated, and they started cursing and gesturing at me. The skinny one kept yelling, "Shut up! Shut up!"

Finally, I said, "Ok, that's it. You asked, and I told you. Nothing more to say."

The big guy said, "Fuck you!" Then they revved up their ride and weaved back and forth down the trail bumping into snowbanks and bushes along the way.

Fortunately, the rest of the night was uneventful, and I was finally able to wind down and get some sleep. When I woke up, I gathered myself and headed out on the trail. About a quarter of a mile away, I saw a snowmobile smashed into pieces alongside a tree, metal fragments slicing into the snow and ice several yards away from the crash. What I surmised was that the larger guy who rode on the back had wrecked his snowmobile and was riding with his buddy to get help. It was no wonder they were so worked up, and of course the alcohol only magnified the situation.

That was one of those bizarre situations that would seem ludicrous anywhere else, but in the wilds of Alaska, you have to be cautious about encounters with strangers. That's why I was always careful about mentioning money or paying for something out in the open. If those guys on the snow mobile had any idea that I was carrying cash, things might have gone a different way. I was traveling on foot, so it would be days before I'd see anyone who might be able to assist; and even then, there would be little they could do.

I was happy to finally reach McGrath, which was 350 miles in. That checkpoint was someone's home and there were no dedicated rooms, just a large gathering area. That was a tough stop because it was located at the end of the most popular race, the 350. Understandably, those racers were celebrating, drinking beer, and comparing notes of the race that they had just completed.

The few of us who were going on to Nome were just in the way because with 650 miles to go, we were in no mood to celebrate. We just wanted to regroup and get back on the trail. It was hard for me to stay focused and in the right frame of mind when everyone else was partying and talking about going home. That was about one-third of the way through the 1,000, and it was tricky because you could easily get caught up in the revelry and hastily decide to pack it in.

I had to get in and get out as quick as I could. I didn't want to allow myself to get comfortable because that would throw me off my game and I couldn't risk that. I had to stay in competitor mode. After that checkpoint, there were no more lodges. One of the places was actually a school that allowed us to sleep on the gymnasium floor. It looked like a comfortable place to get out of the weather, and I was excited to get there until I went inside. In the gym were at least 35 smelly mushers from the Iditarod dogsled race spread out and snoring away, their barking dogs not far away. That was one of those times when I chose to sleep outside because it was a better way for me to rest up while maintaining my concentration.

There were a few times when I'd been hiking through the night and caught myself nodding off while I was still walking. A bush or tree branch would graze my shoulder and snap me awake. I found that I could cover a couple of miles that way before it became too dangerous. It was a strange sensation, but I was pushing myself to the limit and was determined not to give in to sleep unless absolutely necessary.

If I happened upon a rustic lean-to that barely kept out the wind, I'd jump at the chance to at least close my eyes for a few hours. Once I was ready to settle down, the challenge was to fall asleep because it was so cold that it took time for my body to acclimate. I could not remove my gloves because my hands would freeze. I'd also learned not to take off my shoes because they could freeze and then be impossible to get back on. If you tried to dry them in your sleeping bag, they would become wet and practically useless. Then there were times that I was shaking so hard to stay warm that it prevented me from going to sleep.

When I was forced to sleep outside, I would have to get out my mat first because I couldn't lie directly on the snow. Then I'd get my sleeping bag and try to blow up the pad if the nozzle wasn't frozen solid. Or I'd try to heat some water to thaw the nozzle. One thing would lead to another, and it became a vicious cycle that only served to waste time, searching for elusive comfort. Even if I were able to fall asleep, I'd get so cold that it was clear the only way to warm up was to keep moving. That meant I'd have to carefully re-pack everything back into the sled and get back on the trail in hopes of a better resting spot.

On a nice day, meaning 20 degrees above zero, I would put on as many layers as I needed and literally fall into the brush and go to sleep. I wouldn't even waste time with a sleeping bag. It was so much more efficient to just burrow down into the snow for a quick snooze. It wouldn't last long because the involuntary shivering would wake me, and I'd be back on the trail again. At least it afforded me an hour or so of sleep.

Another benefit of the checkpoints was that some allowed racers to receive packages. They would mail themselves a food drop so they wouldn't have to transport it during the race. Naturally, it was all about the logistics because out in the Alaskan wilderness, services aren't quite as reliable as they might be elsewhere.

The other option was to mail something to the town post office and mark it as general delivery. Then you could pick it up as you arrived in town. When that worked out, it was a great way to get a much-needed boost from new supplies. However, if your calculations were off and you passed through that town at night or on a Friday, the post office might not re-open until 9:00 a.m. on Monday. Then you're faced with another decision. Do you wait and lose a few days of travel to get that bounty of food, or do you forget about it and keep going?

Tough choice for some, but that answer was easy for me. I'm so competitive that I would not be able to idle for that long. Wasting two days of a race waiting on a package was not smart for my game. Plus, there was always the chance that the package could get lost and then that time waiting was for nothing.

Another option was to buy supplies at the local stores. I brought cash with me because I knew that money was the universal language in Alaska. When I lived there, I could get just about anything done if I offered up some cash. However, for those who were inexperienced in dealing with the locals, some could be intimidating. We were on their turf and seen as little more than brash athletes traveling through their town.

I knew enough to be cautious because there were always a few who wouldn't mind causing a little trouble. Those who were inebriated could be scary to deal with. I had been in a handful of situations where things could have come unraveled if given the chance.

I had a guy follow about two feet behind me all the way into a town screaming at me that I owed him money and I needed to buy things for him. I had a tight grip on my trekking pole in case he got any closer. I sure as hell wasn't afraid to protect myself if necessary. Some of the folks there are in dire financial situations and that makes people unpredictable. It's like the wild west there, and rules that are followed elsewhere may mean nothing to them.

Athletes are in a difficult spot because cash is necessary since many places don't have the ability to take a credit card. If you're caught in a tough spot without any money, it can be dangerous. However, carrying a lot of cash around was not a wise move either. It was tricky finding the balance and being discreet when it came to money.

In fact, there was one checkpoint where it cost $250 for one night and it included dinner and breakfast the next morning. I gladly paid it because I needed to get out of the weather, but if I had not had cash on me, I would have been out of luck. The race was a way for them to make money so they would take it as far as they could. For one of those expensive rooms, even if there were two beds, I couldn't allow another racer to take a rest. That would cost another $250. Even using the warm water cost $10 or so. It's their water, their electricity, and their food, so racers have to pay up if they want it.

In one of the cabins, I met an older woman who ran the place, and she was amazing. Her generous spirit really boosted my morale and reminded me that most of the people in that area enjoy sharing their homes and their knowledge with visitors. I had such a good time there with her and her family that it made me sad because I knew that was my last hurrah. Regardless of the outcome, I wasn't going to put myself through another grueling ITI. That meant I would not see her on my travels the way many of the regulars did. Before I left, I told her how grateful I was for her hospitality, and I left a big tip to let her know how much her kindness meant to me.

Being so isolated, there's no getting around how expensive it is, especially for the tourists. At one of the stops, I ordered a dinner that was $130, and it wasn't a Ruth's Chris Steak House. It was a simple but tasty home cooked meal. I was surprised that a couple of places had moved to credit cards, but they were scarce, and cash was always better.

Out on those long, lonesome, quiet trails, things could get a little strange, especially when it was dark. My senses were always heightened, and I knew to stay as alert as possible because nature was beautifully unpredictable. Sometimes, I'd hear something and spend what seemed like hours wondering if it was far away or close by. Sound had a way of reverberating and bouncing off the snow and ice. Pinpointing its direction was tricky.

Sometimes I'd see something move in my peripheral vision and get startled because I wasn't expecting it. It was easy for me to get used to the quiet and loneliness so seeing an animal in that frigid weather was always a shock, even though I was intruding on their terrain. Then I'd discover it was only a squirrel. At night, when things settled down, I'd be woken by the sound of wolves howling. Again, I'd try to decide if they were far enough away that I could go back to sleep. Sometimes, I'd settle on staying up for a bit just to make sure they weren't too close. I wasn't too worried about being in danger, but I didn't want them to happen upon me and become startled.

During those long treks on the trail, the monotony of travel would lull me into a sort of daze where I would hallucinate that I was seeing an animal or even another racer who was not actually there. In that middle ground between light and dark, alert and tired, focused and distracted, my mind would play tricks on me. The rhythmic crunch of snow, the metal runners of the sled slicing through the top layer of ice, my breathing matching pace with my steps. The sounds sometimes crashed together, but other times they fell into sync, finding a melodic harmony that could lull me into a delirious state of mind.

I'd find myself having conversations with someone I thought was right beside me. At times, I'd argue passionately about a point I was trying to make, or I'd argue about something that felt so real. At one point, I was hiking down a hill and saw the deceptively beautiful ocean below. I was excited to reach it, to get near the crashing waves. My plan was to take some time and just let the roiling waters rise and fall. I quickly picked up my pace to reach the bottom of the hill.

Once I made it, I looked down. There were no foamy white waves waiting to greet me. I'd been hiking for three hours to reach yet another frozen body of water. I'd seen beautiful blue waves dancing along the surface, but this reality was much different. My mind was playing tricks on me. It was probably an arctic mirage caused by the extreme atmospheric conditions. Of course, being mentally and physically exhausted only magnified the situation.

With all of those distractions taunting me, it often wasn't the physical stamina that I had to worry about. It was the emotional toll that I had to power through. It took focus and a concerted effort for me to push the mirages and hallucinations and rowdy locals out of my mind so that I could focus. I had to keep reminding myself that the goal was not just to complete the 1,000-mile journey, but to do it first. I understood that it was unlikely because there were other competitors with more experience. But I had to admit to myself that I still visualized it. I desperately wanted my last attempt to end with a first-place win. There was no doubt that it was a long shot, but I had a solid history of betting on myself. This time was no different.

At one point, there was another racer who was truly amazing. I'd been impressed with his performance over the years. However, he had the habit of "correcting" me on my techniques and giving me unsolicited input on how I should be racing. Maybe it was coming from a good place, but it was wearing on me. *Focus on yourself, man. I know what I'm doing!* We were racing close together and even our strides were similar, which meant we would probably be jockeying for position most of the way to Nome. Since Tim was in the race, I figured the two of us were competing for second and third with Tim far in the lead.

My focus was on the finish line. My plan was simple. Do my best, trust my instincts, and finish the 1,000. Having two superstar athletes in the mix only helped fuel my competitive spirit. As we continued, I moved ahead and gained a good amount of distance between us. When the weather changed, I settled down for the night and organized my gear. In the morning, my challenger was in his sleeping bag right beside me!

I said, "I lost sight of you last night. I thought you went ahead without stopping here."

He replied, "It was terrible weather. Why would I do that? Do you think I'm stupid?"

Can't people just answer a simple question or make small talk? Come on. I didn't call him out on it. I just needed to get back on the trail and haul ass. I headed to the main lodge to eat, pack up, and hit the trail.

The folks who ran the lodge were nice enough, but they had a way of making us ITI racers feel like we were intruding. I went in and was wary, but I took the meal they gave me and tried to ignore the attitude. I had just started to suit back up when the other racer walked in.

"Why are you wearing so many layers?" he said, instead of *hello.*

"Hey, stop telling me what to do. I don't need a mother out here. I'm doing my own thing, and you don't need to worry about it."

"Wow, someone woke up in a rough mood."

"That's right. I'm in a rough mood, and I'm tired of you talking to me like that."

"OK," he said.

Other racers in the cabin watched our exchange without chiming in. My competitive spirit mixed with strong independence meant I wasn't allowing any abuse this time. I was taking a stand when I needed to and showing everyone that I was a serious contender.

Later, we were both on the trail, once again neck and neck, until he veered off without realizing it. I kept moving straight ahead until I saw a different racer heading toward me with his headlamp shining in the twilight.

"What are you doing?" I asked.

"I'm heading to the checkpoint."

"No," I said. "That's the wrong direction."

He said, "No, it's on my GPS. You are going the wrong way."

I can tell you there are a few advantages to doing the race so many times. I sure as hell knew where the checkpoints were. Those were like our lifelines, and you tend to remember their locations. Just then, I turned around and saw that my competitor had already realized he had made a mistake. He had gotten turned around trying to find the main Iditarod Trail. When we met up later, I knew that he'd screwed up, and he knew that I knew.

Finally, he broke the silence. "I know I made a mistake."

I smiled. "No big deal, man. I'm doing me. I'm not leaning on you to get me through this. Let's just do our own thing. "

Any little event could either derail racers out on the trail or fuel them to continue. When he came at me in that cabin, it only made me more determined to finish before him. I had nothing to lose and everything to gain by just going all out. At one point as we kept running into each other, he said, "I'd rather be alone on the trail." That was cool with me.

My brother Scott was tracking me, and I put in a call to him on my satellite phone. He acted as my eyes for the overall race and gave me info on the others. "How am I doing?" I asked him. My personal goal was to try and stay within 24 hours of superstar Tim because I knew he'd likely lead the way the entire time and cross the finish line a full day before me. So, I asked, "Where's Tim in the race? How far ahead?" I needed to know.

Scott's voice vibrated through the phone. "Tim quit."

Chapter Thirteen

The Journey

Having Scott as my lifeline was invaluable, not only in 2018 but the other trips as well. He talked me through my perilous journey just before I took the icy plunge into the Tatiana. I'd clung to him as my eyes on the trail, a way to see through the snowstorms and beyond the towering mountains. He told me how he continually refreshed the online tracker to keep me on his radar when he couldn't reach me by phone. Along with the rest of my family and friends, he was following my every move, wondering if I was safe and if I was making the right decisions.

This time, he'd come through once again and we talked almost daily about how I was progressing and where I was on the trail. I'd call him and say, "Man, I'm lost. Can you check it out?" and he'd rush to his computer or phone and guide me back. One time, I called him, and I was at my breaking point. "Scott, I'm freezing, frustrated, and miserable. I can't get my bearings, and it's just too much, man. I can't finish."

"Pete, look at it this way. If you're at your lowest point now, that's a good thing because the only way you can go is up, right? Right?"

"Yeah, I guess," I said.

"Hey, it's your decision. You can either have a fucking pity party, or you can stay on that trail and get your ass moving. I know you can do it. Finish on your own terms."

I loved how he was real with me and not just trying to make me feel better. He was helping to motivate me. I really appreciated it, too, because being that support system and doing that tracking was a full-time job during the race. It was a lot of stress, and I never took that dedication for granted.

So, when he gave me that news, I knew he wasn't bullshitting. Still, it was hard to comprehend. "Tim did not quit. He doesn't quit," I told Scott over the phone. "Tim's done this race 10 times. He always finishes, and he usually wins!"

"Well, I'm watching his tracker go south on the Yukon River, not north along the trail."

"Did he make a wrong turn? That's not like him."

A little later, Scott called back. "They sent out word that Tim turned in his tracker and officially quit when he got to Anchorage."

I couldn't believe it. I was stunned.

"Pete, listen to me. You're leading the Iditarod Trail Invitational right now!"

I turned to see my competitor right beside me. I hung up the phone and said, "Big news. Tim quit."

"Yeah, I overheard your call, but I don't believe it. Something's not right."

"It's true. He's off the trail and back in Anchorage."

We were about 600 miles in and there was only one other racer on the trail besides us, but he was much farther behind. We looked at each other, realizing that first place was up for grabs. Until that point, I had thought we'd basically travel together and finish around the same time. We had finally started to get along better anyway. I'd begun to understand him and realized his responses were curt but not malicious. He just had a different delivery than I was used to. With a few hundred miles left to go, it was going to be a fight to the finish. I didn't want to just tie the race anymore. I wanted to win.

The news about Tim was exciting, but it didn't really change anything as far as my day-to-day except for the reality that one of us was going to win and neither of us had ever won before. I hadn't even completed a 1,000 yet. So, it was a pretty exciting opportunity for both of us, the reality of the situation finally sinking in.

Part of the trail required crossing a huge body of water far more treacherous and intimidating than the Tatina. Because of its size, there were many more opportunities for compromised ice. However, that was the only way to reach the all-important checkpoint that served as a food drop for the racers. The rest of the way to the finish line was all hard trail work.

Finally reaching that checkpoint was a real boost for me because I needed to take a breather and refuel. Cautiously negotiating the slick ice had taken a lot out of me. Once inside, the woman there told me two things: first, I smelled bad. (*No kidding, lady.*) Second, there was no box with my name on it.

Ignoring the first comment, I replied, "It has to be here. I need it. There's no way I can go on without it. Can you check again?"

She checked again and confirmed that there were "no packages for Pete Ripmaster." "This is not good," I said aloud as my mind raced. What was I going to do? I saw they had a tiny store run by the locals that carried things like animal crackers and old, dry pasta.

Then she said, "We do have some boxes that were sent for racers who have already dropped out."

I knew they wouldn't mind helping out a fellow athlete and the woman said it was OK, so I rummaged through and grabbed anything that looked like it might be decent fuel for the remainder of the race. I pushed on and kept moving at a good clip but felt defeated because I didn't have everything I'd planned to use. The ITI, and any ultra-event for that matter, required as much planning as possible. When my plans fell through, the plans I'd been counting on, it shook my concentration.

I called my brother on the satellite phone the next morning. I knew that the food had been sent. "Scott, would you do me a favor and just call the post office to ask them to look one more time to see if a box is there for Ripmaster? And if so, I'm going to need somebody from that town to get on a snowmobile and bring it out to me. Tell them it's worth $100 cash if someone can do that."

When Scott called back and said they found the package, I was relieved, but still irritated by the mistake. You've gotta be kidding me! Of course, in those small towns, things can easily go awry. I knew it was important to be adaptable, but that was hard to do when I was miserable and starving.

Back on the trail, I dug in my trekking poles with each step. Stab, slide, stab, slide. It was arduous and really began to take its toll. Then, without any warning, I was in a whiteout. A flurry of snow and wind whipped around me with surprising force. I couldn't believe my bad luck. How would my supplies make it in this weather?

To keep my mind occupied, I tried every trick I could think of. I used my numbering system. I estimated how far I'd gone and even tried to calculate how many steps I'd taken. Anything to stay focused and keep my mind from wandering into dangerous territory. I also dug deep and tried to convince myself that the supplies didn't matter. I could make it no matter what.

Just then I saw two fluorescent lights bounding up the hill in the snowstorm. It was a guy with my supplies! Holy shit, I couldn't believe he'd made it. Having that feeling of elation come flooding in gave me the mental boost I needed.

"You must be Peter," the guy yelled.

"Yes!" To verify it, I pulled out a crisp C-note and gave it to him. He smiled and presented me with the most beautiful cardboard box I'd ever seen. It was as if I'd been given a treasure chest; it was that precious to me and my mental focus. I hastily pulled out a knife, slashed open the box, and emptied the contents onto the frozen snow. I still had a lot of work ahead of me, but this sign of hope would help my performance on the trail.

By the time I reached the next pit stop, I was exhausted and struggling to stay motivated. Even with the bounty of food, going 1,000 miles was much more difficult than I had anticipated. The next checkpoint was basically a shelter cabin with a wood-burning stove. The wind whistled through loose floorboards and the stove struggled to provide heat, but it was better than being out in the elements.

It was around 3:00 a.m., so I started my meal and stepped out on the rickety deck to answer nature's call. Typically, there's no one for miles and miles, but I saw a snowmobile pull up. At first, I thought it was a mirage.

"Hey, are you alright?" the guy yelled.

"Yes," I assured him. "I'm in the ITI, but it's slow going. To be honest, it's brutal."

"How can I help?"

"If you'd just hang out here for a few minutes, that would be awesome," I told him.

I was glad that I'd managed to get the inside temperature of the cabin up, but my new friend was taken aback. "Whoa, it's warm in here." As a native Alaskan, I'm sure he was used to much cooler temperatures, even inside.

"Maybe I used a little too much wood," I said sheepishly.

We both sat down, and he was incredibly compassionate. He told me he was a whale hunter and the elder in his town. He was in his mid-fifties and had a large family with lots of kids. I could hear the pride in his voice as this tough mountain man talked about how important his village and his family were to him. He was so kind and generous that we ended up talking for a couple of hours. I felt so comfortable that I just shared with him. I told him about how I'd struggled losing my parents, the difficulties I'd had finding my place in the world, and how much racing meant to me, even though the 1,000 was kicking my ass.

He said, "The next checkpoint is my village. I want you to come to my house. I want to show you our Alaskan hospitality."

"Oh, you have no idea how much that would mean to me," I said with a smile.

Arriving at the next station, I was met by two young boys playing in the yard.

"Are you Pete?" one of them asked.

Once I confirmed, they led me to their cozy house. Inside was a large family ready to greet me. I began removing some of my layers and apologized for how dirty I was.

A woman said, "If you change clothes, we can quickly take care of your laundry while you eat."

She motioned to the table, and there was an amazing bounty of caribou, salmon, rice, and many other dishes waiting to be explored. After subsisting on power bars, gummy bears, and granola, the beer and fish provided my body with much-needed fuel. The caribou was amazing, and I devoured every bit on my plate. I couldn't believe the generosity and warmth they showed a complete stranger, but I welcomed it.

Soon, I packed the clean clothes in my bag and thanked them for their graciousness. That extension of hospitality and genuine concern helped motivate me even more than the meal. It was my soul and my spirit that had been depleted, and that pit stop was just what I'd needed.

I made sure to find the right trail and continued the next 25 miles to the next checkpoint. I was surprised to see my new friend waiting for me on his snowmobile.

"Hey, Pete, just wanted to make sure you were OK," my guardian angel Eric said before zooming off in a white cloud of snow.

That encounter was so fortuitous and coincided with my own inner work on staying mindful, grateful, and present. With all the alone time on the trail, I'd focused on being aware of my mental and spiritual state. My goal was to build that foundation of being in the moment and in touch with my thoughts, feelings, and emotions, as well as my physical well-being. All those elements needed to work together, especially in an endurance race.

It was at that point, as I continued my self-work on the trail, that I reflected on ego and self-importance and how to separate that from my conscious reality. I began to understand that my identity was much deeper and more complex than I'd realized. There was more to life than striving for accolades and awards. It may sound trite, but that mindfulness helped me place the importance where it belonged: on continuing to develop my spirit and learning to enjoy the moment. We are taught from a young age that the goal is to be the best, to win, and that's when we will find satisfaction.

That is where I continually found issues when I played team sports, went to school, and even worked various jobs. Everything was about the motivation to keep striving for something that could never be attained. One win on the field meant winning again and again. School was centered around tests and semester grades and GPAs. Teaching was about meeting metrics and striving for a yearly raise.

I could see that it was an endless cycle of punishment and reward that I had been taught since childhood as the only way to live. The problem was that I never found that satisfaction, and I realized that being self-centered and striving to always be the best did not fulfill me. It was hilarious to me that at around 850 miles into a 1,000-mile race, I was performing my own self-therapy as I strived to finish first in the toughest endurance race in the world. I came to the realization that I got all my inner fuel from the journey, interacting with the wildlife, paying respect to the majestic surroundings, and meeting locals like that gracious family. That's the importance of the experience, and to my understanding that was the real prize.

Taking stock of my life and prioritizing what is important made all the difference. Along my journey, I was able to celebrate the people in my life, my grandma who always stands by me, my siblings, and my wife and girls. The truth was that I didn't need to fit the mold of what I should be in order to be happy. That mindfulness helped me realize that I could be myself, and that was enough. I could be introspective, goofy, intense, loving, and competitive in my own way, the way that worked for me.

To some, it might seem like a small victory, but to a guy like me who has suffered incredibly tough times and dealt with crippling depression and self-doubt all my life, it was nothing short of life changing. The experience out on that trail led me to a new level of inner peace and self-worth. Winning was not the only goal-- it was part of it--but for me, the real win was learning to value and treasure the entire experience. The journey was the gift.

That realization shocked me into a new reality in which I was able to understand that all the other times that I'd competed in the ITI and any other race, it was only to win. Understanding that winning wasn't enough was a true breakthrough. It was important for me to enjoy and celebrate the entire experience—the good and bad. When I did that, the finish would be much more meaningful. That motivated me more than first place.

At that point, I was starving for some fuel to finish the race strong. As I reached one of the few remaining checkpoints, I remembered back to when I was packing back home in Asheville. Kristen said, "What is one food that you'd really like on the trail?"

I was in my warm house thinking about good food and said, "I really like spicy beef jerky."

Now only a few dozen miles away from the finish line, the inside of my mouth was covered with open sores from the crap I had been eating. I also hadn't taken enough care of my health, including my mouth. It was like a crazy Petri dish in there, and it ached with every cold breath I sucked in. If I tried to eat anything that was even slightly salty, it was like my mouth was on fire.

I couldn't wait to see what kind of awesome food was in my box. I slowly opened it and peeked inside. There were seven bags filled with various types of spicy beef jerky, each one hotter and spicier than the next. I was going to just toss them or leave them for someone else because there was no way I could down one of those at that point.

Then I dug down into the box and at the bottom were two bags of candy—Swedish Fish and sour gummy bears. I knew that was the work of my daughter, Reagan. She and I both share a love of sweets, and I knew she had tossed a couple of bags of candy in there for me. I had to throw out about 95% of the box, but that candy was like gold to me, and it would have to sustain me for the final 50 miles.

I continued to trudge along, and when I was about 980 miles in, I was surrounded by a few bike riders because the conditions were so tough that they were actually slower than I was. We all made it to the final checkpoint, and we were sitting outside because it was closed. We were jazzed about finishing the race soon, so I stayed for a bit and then declared that I was ready to get back on the trail.

As I started to make my way, I realized that I hadn't seen my footrace competitor for about 50 miles, so I wasn't sure of his location, and I hadn't really thought about it. My plan was that, after realigning my goals to focus on the journey, I still wanted to finish strong to complete the process. I'd already won an internal battle as far as I was concerned, so anything else would be gravy.

That's when I heard the bikers behind me yelling and gesturing. *OK, I get it, you guys want me to slow down, but I'm keeping my focus. Sorry, gotta keep moving.* What they were trying to tell me was that I'd inadvertently gotten on the dogsled trail, not the ITI route, and added five bonus miles to the trip! Damn. It was not the time to make a costly mistake like that, but I changed course and made up the time I'd lost.

I picked up the pace as best I could because I knew the end had to be near. Finally, I saw faraway lights flickering along the horizon line. I realized that beautiful light was coming from the Nome airport located on the outskirts of the town. The finish line was in sight! It was overwhelming to think that I had covered 1,000 miles in the treacherous snow and ice of an Alaskan winter. It was difficult to process the fact that it was almost over. That I had done what I'd set out to do, and from the looks of it, I was the first one to make it. Amazing!

Soon, I was walking on the concrete of the airport tarmac with less than five miles to go. Then I saw a truck driving around in circles, and I thought, *don't come near me!* I was so close that I didn't need anything to interfere with my progress. No surprises! Then I realized it was my friend who had come to see me finish the race. He'd been following my tracker and knew that I was so close! That gave me the extra shot of adrenaline I needed.

When I reached the sleepy Main Street of Nome, I saw there were no teeming crowds waiting to greet the finishers. Then I checked the time. 4:00 a.m. No wonder. I did see one of my fellow racers who had recently finished on his bike. He was standing with a lady who was filming me as I crossed the finish line. They congratulated me and yelled, "Pete, you just won first place in the Iditarod! You're the winner! You did it!" It was a modest welcoming committee for sure, but I'd take it!

"Yee-haw!" I shouted as I gave a wave.

While I'd been able to reconnect with myself emotionally along the trail, my body had taken a beating. I'd started the race at a healthy 210, but by the end, I had lost about 40 pounds. I felt sick and completely devoid of energy. I pushed my body to its limit and that had sucked everything out of me.

I later found out that part of the reason I felt so lethargic was that I'd contracted Giardia, which was a fairly common ailment among survivalists. Giardia is a type of parasite that is transported through contaminated food or water or areas with poor sanitation.

One of the unpleasant aspects of the ITI (and many endurance events) was that because it lasted so long and the checkpoints often had no modern plumbing, the surrounding area could become contaminated with waste. The illness can then spread to anyone who comes in contact with the same area, and it was nasty to say the least. Enduring all those obstacles—mental, emotional, and now physical—was so much more draining than I'd anticipated.

It may have been more evident to me because I'd started the race with one mindset and finished with a totally new way of thinking. I'd used those days and nights of unending solitude to make some meaningful changes in my life. I'd been able to focus so much on self-care that I'd pushed through the physical pain without realizing what a toll it was taking on my body.

All the competitors who completed the race were put up in a hotel, and the next day was filled with interviews, pictures, and social media posts. It was surreal and overwhelming. Part of that was due to my growth. Where I'd normally have boasted and celebrated, I found myself more reserved and grateful without being arrogant. But I was struggling physically. On one hand, I wanted to give them what they needed to hear and play the part of the winner; but on the other hand, I just wanted to throw up and go to bed.

One of my thoughts during the race, one of the things that helped motivate me, was fantasizing about what my first meal would be once I'd crossed that finish line. Finally, I decided I was just going to the closest restaurant and ordering one of everything on the menu. And I did just that.

The odd thing was that I couldn't eat much of it. I sat and stared at the bounty before me, and it was sensory overload. After subsisting on so little, it was too much too soon. I didn't even know how to go about eating so much food. In my mind, it was the right thing to do, load up on the sustenance that I'd denied myself for so long, but my body rebelled. I needed to heal first.

For weeks I'd eaten mostly what I called crap food or space-ship food. I liked convenient, easy-to-eat, prepackaged snacks that I could down on the go. I liked to think of it as quick nutrition. It didn't need to taste good. I'd just stuff it in my mouth and go. As long as it had at least 200 calories, I was good.

I'd started out eating nutritious foods like energy chews and power bars. That lasted while I was on the trail, but once I reached a checkpoint with food, I'd order anything—pizza, fries, Snickers bars—I just needed the calories. If there were leftovers, I'd pack them up and save them for later.

During the flight from Anchorage to North Carolina, I felt even worse and kept going to the restroom. I couldn't get comfortable, I was sweating like crazy, and I just wanted it to be over. The man in the seat beside me just shook his head and said, "What's wrong with you?"

Dude, you have no idea!

At my layover in Atlanta, I was reading social media and one of the posts caught my eye. *Hey, I hope everyone knows about the hero's welcome that we're going to have at the airport for Pete.* Holy hell! It's not that I wasn't appreciative, but when you're that sick and uncomfortable, the last thing you want is a freaking audience.

Upon arrival in Asheville, around 40 people were waiting to greet me along with local media lights and cameras. Kids were holding up balloons and homemade signs just waiting to explode with applause when they saw their newly crowned hometown hero. Seeing my wife and the kids gave me a small burst of energy. I was able to power through the interviews and smile for photos.

After getting settled back in at home, I had to go to the doctor twice a day to have intravenous fluids administered. Physically, it took several months before I started feeling somewhat back to normal. It made me wonder how people like Tim could compete in that race 10 times or more. Maybe others can withstand it better than I could; I'm not sure. All I know is that the punishment to your body can affect your health for the rest of your life.

But it was my dream, and at 42 years old, I achieved it. I'd been thinking about it for as long as I could remember, then I'd wormed my way into the 2014 race and went back every year until finally winning in 2018. When I set that goal, I knew it would be insanely difficult, but the reality of it was beyond my comprehension. Still, despite all of that, I was happy that I'd not only completed the race, but I had also won—and on *my* terms.

Being back at home and falling into the old routine was a little tricky. After all the craziness I'd been through, I found myself driving the girls to school and sitting in the car line along with 75 suburban mothers in Grand Caravans and Chevy Tahoes. It felt a little strange and jarring to go from such intensity to everyday life. Adjusting, or readjusting, was not as easy as I'd thought it would be. Not to mention the fact that people would come up to me and ask personal questions because I looked so weak.

"Wow, are you OK? Are you ill?"

"No," I'd respond. "I won the 1,000-mile ITI race."

There were plenty of good things that came out of the experience. I received a lot of attention and this time, not only locally, but nationally and even internationally. The ITI 1,000 is one of the ultimate physical challenges, so athletes around the world follow it each year. I did a lot of interviews and camera appearances while working to maintain my authenticity and be as real as possible. Winning the ITI also made me more in demand on the speaking circuit. I was contacted by corporations, fitness organizations, and schools to talk about the experience.

Each time I agreed to one of those events, I was careful to remind them that I am the real deal. What you see is what you get with me: a cowboy hat, my favorite boots, and sheer positivity. My message always focuses on applying yourself, remembering that life is mental as well as physical, and understanding that everything is more rewarding when you are happy with yourself. I tell them about the struggles I've gone through and what has worked for me, how it's taken me decades to realize my true potential, and how they can work to achieve their own happiness.

The first thing I do at any speaking gig is to ask how many have heard of the Iditarod. There is usually a decent number. Then I ask how many have heard of the Iditarod Trail Invitational. Typically, very few. That helps me establish a baseline with the audience. I know how much background I need to give to set the stage for my crazy Alaskan adventure.

Some events are amazing experiences where folks leave with a feeling of positivity and goodwill. Others are not so successful. As a favor, I spoke at a certain college, but I didn't have a lot of details about the event. When I arrived, I found out that the auditorium was filled with more than 500 fraternity students. That wasn't what I'd expected, but I can pivot with the best of them. I tried my jokes and stories, but they were not landing with these teenagers. As I showed the slides and told my tales, I could see them falling asleep or poking each other or looking at their phones. It was tough to stay focused, but I did. Not too long ago, I would have been devastated by something like that, but this time I understood my audience, withheld judgment, and did my best.

One of my speaking events was a corporate retreat at a fancy resort and spa in Pennsylvania. When I checked into the hotel, I was greeted at the door.

"Mr. Ripmaster?"

"How did you know it was me?" I asked.

"We've been waiting for your arrival. Do you need help with your bags?"

"No," I assured him, "I'm fine. Which way is my room?"

"Please wait here. Your butler will be down momentarily to collect your bag and show you to your room."

"Oh, no, can you just give me the key?"

The lady at the desk motioned for me to come over, "Sir, you are going to have to let yourself be pampered for a couple of days. That's what we do here."

"OK, OK," I said as I held up my hands in surrender.

After I was settled in my room, my butler insisted that I let him know when I needed anything. That's what he was there for. Just call. So, I took the time to get comfortable, smoked a joint and relaxed. Then I noticed a menu by the soaking tub. It listed different types of baths that could be requested. What the hell? I called my butler and told him what I wanted.

As promised, the butler was there in no time. "Mr. Ripmaster, I need to prepare your bath."

"Uh, sure," I said as I stepped aside.

I could hear him rustling around in there, and he soon came out. "Mr. Ripmaster, your Rose Petal bath experience awaits."

Poking my head in the bathroom, I saw that the tub was filled with scented water, rose petals were strewn around on the floor, and candles flickered with the suggestion of a romantic evening. I had no idea I had chosen the romantic package. It was hilarious, and I laughed like a crazy man as I lowered myself into the most amazing bath I'd ever had.

While winning the ITI was one of my life goals, I certainly couldn't stop there. Life is all about new experiences. So, my follow-up challenge is a long-term project that will take at least the next 10 years to complete. I've taken the 50 marathons in 50 states challenge one step further by upping the ante. I've committed to running a 100-mile run/race in all 50 states.

Besides proving to myself that I can do it, the primary goal is to raise money for an important environmental nonprofit. The Owl Research Institute is dedicated to owl research, conservation, and education. In all my experience with creatures throughout my life, owls have held a special meaning and spiritual significance. If there is a way that I can possibly give back to them and their preservation, now is the time to do it. My goal is to raise at least $50,000 for this worthy cause.

Using my website and social media, I've begun the arduous journey of fulfilling my next challenge; and this time, taking with me all I've learned, I'm able to do it on my own terms. I bring my family when it's possible, and I'm enjoying the process. In the past, there were times when I felt like I was doing what was expected of me. This time, it is more personal.

The ITI victory has given me the ability to step back and see things differently, but that didn't come from the win, it came from the journey. It came from the work I was able to do on myself. The sweetest reward is often the unexpected one, and that's exactly how it happened for me.

Winning the Iditarod Trail Invitational took me 42 years, but what I got out of it will last a lifetime.

Epilogue

It's still a joy to celebrate my successes with family, especially my grandmother. Our bond remains strong. Going through the loss of my mother and my grandmother's husband, we leaned on each other to get through the heartbreak.

In the hospital room before they removed her life support, I told Mom, "You're going to be proud of me in the future." That was a turning point for me, and my grandmother knew it. She understood that I felt guilt over the crazy stunts I'd pulled and the worry I'd put Mom through.

Later, Grandma told me, "You don't have anything to worry about. I'm sure she is smiling on you from heaven."

When something good happens, I love calling Grandma Dobson to talk about it. Our extended family continues to vacation together and remains involved in each other's lives. When she received an honorary degree from the University of Michigan, I flew up and surprised her.

"Peter, what are you doing here? You didn't have to—"

"Yes, I did. Congratulations!"

When she was awarded the Citizen of the Year award from United Way, I did the same thing. Another reason I value her is that she not only understands my professional choices but my personal ones as well. Not all my relatives were on board when I chose to stay home to raise my daughters. Some thought I should be behind a desk because that's how they were raised, but Grandma's support remained steadfast.

"The way you pick up those girls from school and help with their homework, how you laugh together as a family, it's perfect for you. I know you've had some stumbles, but you've had plenty of successes, and it's all led to the life you have now. Time with your children is something you will never regret."

I'm not sure that she always understood why I took on some of my crazy adventure challenges, but that never dampened her support or enthusiasm. "Being able to appreciate nature is a gift," she said. "Talking to the crows and honoring the owls is a special experience. That's something you'd miss if you were stuck in an office or sitting in traffic. I'm glad you found your own way. Most people are guilty of wishing they'd done something different with their lives, but yours is richer because you've followed your heart."

I still strive to come up with physical challenges that force me to test my limits, and I'm often inspired by nature's serene beauty. During the 2014 Iditarod Trail Invitational, I had a magical encounter with a majestic snowy owl. It left an indelible impression on me, and I've been studying those amazing creatures ever since.

The Owl Run Hundreds Project will take about nine or ten years, but it's my hope that the journey will motivate and inspire others to get involved and lend a hand to a cause that touches their heart, like the Owl Research Institute does for me. This project was even more special because my family helped me launch the event with a video shared on social media.

Having the support not only of my family but friends I've known for years makes some of my outrageous dreams a reality. Speaking to groups, clubs, and company employees took up a lot of my time before the COVID-19 pandemic. I was flying around the country, sometimes to a small sports-oriented business that was promoting the outdoor lifestyle, and other times to a huge corporate event. Regardless of the venue or the number of people in attendance, I always stay true to myself and tell my unfiltered story, warts and all. I've been amazed by how many people have approached me or sent emails saying how I've inspired them or someone in their family.

It also excites me that I've been able to turn the crazy stages of my life into a motivational program that not only uplifts people but inspires them to be unique and follow their own path. People love not only the stories of harrowing challenges like surviving a plunge into a frozen river or facing the punishing Alaskan weather, but also the fact that I didn't give up. It's not that I didn't want to—because a lot of times I did—but having a support system to back me up and a stubborn streak that told me things would be OK got me through some tough spots. Hopefully, others get that message after hearing my tall tales.

The pandemic has slowed my speech commitments, but it will take more than a global virus to stop me. While I continue the Owl Run Hundreds, I also created a company with a couple of buddies, including Haig. He went into the tech industry and now owns a thriving, innovative company. So we've partnered on a project called Rad Endurance. The first event was a virtual Iditarod race where participants could run, walk, bike, or swim the virtual trail from Wasilla to Nome, Alaska. It was a completely virtual event where athletes participated at their own pace, either solo or in a team. I played the role of guide, coach, and motivator for "the raddest race on the planet!"

These projects help channel my manic energy and addictive personality in a positive, productive way. Through these challenges, I'm able to show my girls, and everyone else, that we all have obstacles to overcome and inner voices to manage. Seeing an athlete push through adversity and cross the finish line in the No. 1 position can give an impression of superiority or unwavering confidence. My story shows that it's more about perseverance and positivity. It took a long time, but I eventually learned how to channel my energy, love of nature, and mental challenges into a life that continues to reward me not only with race victories but experiences that I cherish.

In June of 2020, my family wanted to get away and I wasn't going to let the pandemic slow us down. I love showing my daughters the wonders of nature, and I hope they develop a passion for it the way I did. So, we packed up the trusty family Suburban and drove from Asheville, North Carolina, to Telluride, Colorado, with plenty of meetups with friends scheduled along the way. Our western road trip was a dream come true for me, and I couldn't wait to get them to our Ripmaster Ranch to start making memories.

Our first jaunt was about 750 miles through Tennessee, Kentucky, and Illinois to Lake of the Ozarks state park in Missouri. Then we went through Kansas (no tickets this time!), stopped in Lawrence, and landed in Colorado. We drove the final 375 miles from Boulder to Telluride on the third day, and it felt amazing to be back in my spiritual homeland.

Via Ferrata is a mountain-climbing path located in the Alps and the concept has been adapted to many other mountain terrains around the world. The one in Ouray, Colorado, uses a harness and steel cables to guide climbers along the challenging path with makeshift handholds and footings, as a river flows beneath them. The way it works is that there are two safety clips, so if one is unclipped, the other is there for safety. We stressed to Hunter and Reagan that one clip must stay secured at all times. At one point, we were way up on the mountain. I'm not sure about the elevation, but it was high up. Hunter, my oldest daughter, started going sideways. She was hot, sweaty, and exhausted from traversing the steep incline. Kristen and I looked at each other because we both knew Hunter was reaching her limit.

At one point, the instructor told Hunter to remove one of the clips, and the next thing we knew, she had taken them both off. She was standing on a ledge holding one in each of her hands, without the safety of the cable. If she had lost her footing, it would have been over. Before I could say anything, she reached over and casually snapped one clip and then the other on the cable. We immediately changed course and headed back down the mountain.

Seeing my daughter in that situation gave me flashbacks of all the crazy chances I've taken during my climbs, runs, and hikes. When I was in those situations, I had the experience and confidence to know that I'd probably be able to figure my way out of a tough spot. Seeing her in a similar dilemma was eye-opening because it drove home the message that it's not about just me anymore. I have a family to consider; not only for their safety but mine. I can't be as reckless as I once was because I'm not about to leave them without a dad. I have come to terms with the realization that I can continue challenging myself and being immersed in the beauty of nature; there's just a different layer I have to consider. It felt like I'd come full circle by bringing my kids to the place where my dad brought us kids.

Sharing my love of adventure and the importance of appreciating God's beautiful planet is something I teach my girls every day by how I live my life. Whether it's a crazy trip across the country or watching black bears play in the backyard at our mountain home in North Carolina, it's an important part of who I am and it's an honor to pass that on to them. As I tell my girls, adventure calls and we must answer!

Yee-Haw!

Photos

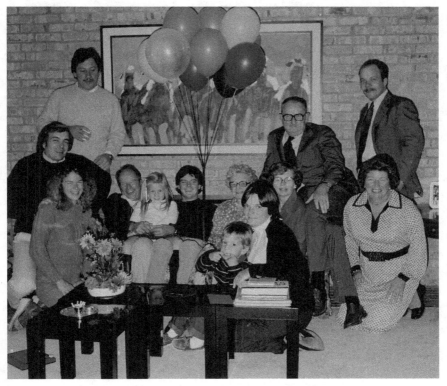

My people! This is an early family picture taken in my
birthplace of Ann Arbor, MI. My mother is holding me in
the front row and as usual, I'm making a sour face which
was the norm for me in all family photos. I've always hated
posed pictures.
Connie Belda

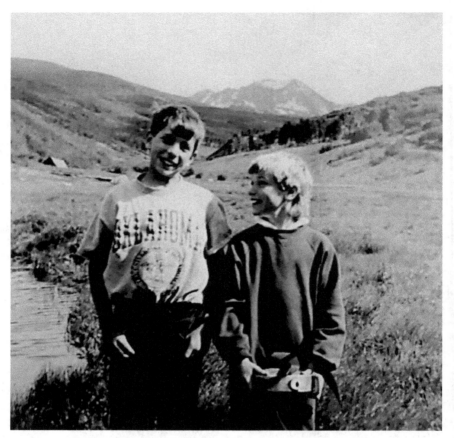

A picture of me and my younger brother Scott on our first western trip to Telluride, CO in 1989. I was twelve in this picture and my dad had decided it was to be a trip of firsts for me; chewing tobacco, tasting whiskey and buying a "Playboy" magazine. This trip opened my eyes on multiple levels and had me dreaming of the west from an early age.

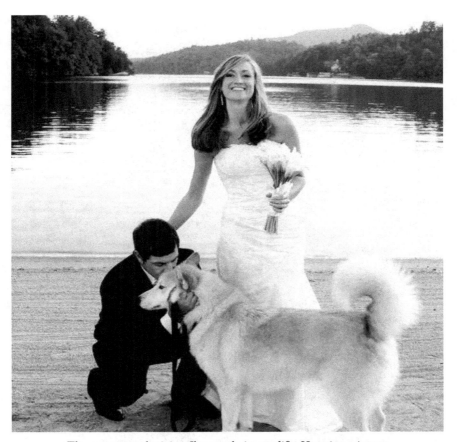

The smartest decision I've made in my life. Here is a picture of me and Kristen on our wedding day. It was a treat to have my wolf hybrid Percy involved in the ceremony. September 30, 2006 was a special day with friends and family in Lake Lure, NC.

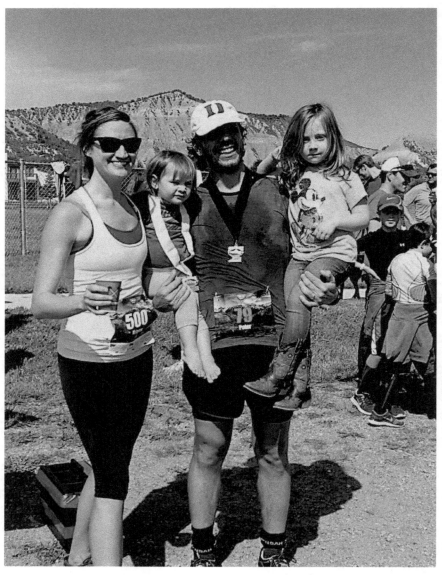

Not long after getting married, I ran my first marathon in 2008. Little did I know that decision would impact my life in a big way, including running 50 marathons in 50 states. Here I am with my wife and little girls after finishing my 50th state, Colorado, of course!

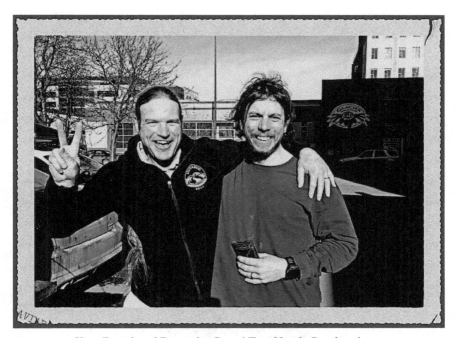

King David and Peter the Great! Two North Carolina boys
with over 5,000 combined miles on foot during the Iditarod
Trail Invitational. Dave Johnston was one of my ITI heroes
before he became one of my best friends. I'll never forget
having this picture taken after finishing my very first ITI in
2014, the beginning of my ITI journey.

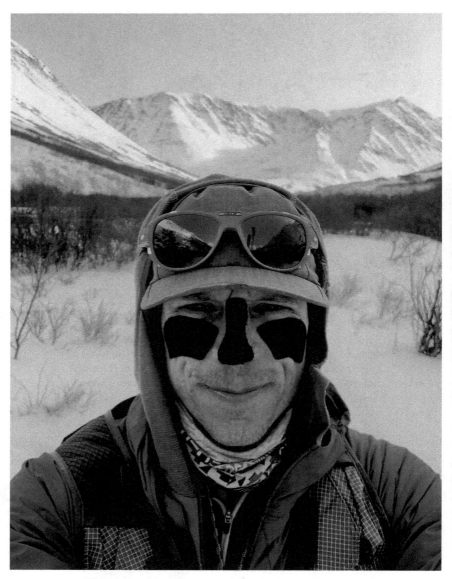

The Iditarod Trail Invitational was my school of hard
knocks. It took years to become comfortable and efficient
in the Alaskan wilderness. With over 2,500 hard-fought
miles on the Iditarod Trail, this is clearly a picture of
confidence and contentment. It never came easy.

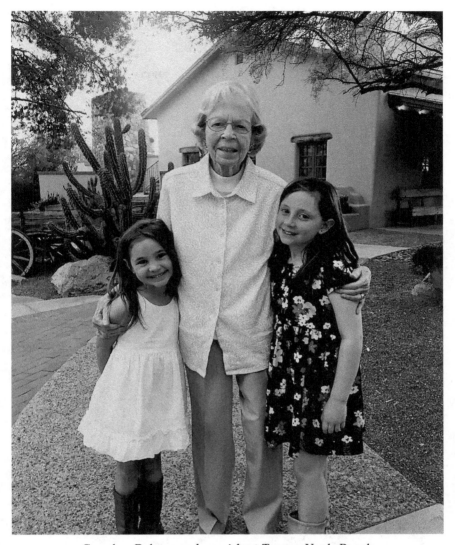

Grandma Dobson and my girls at Tanque Verde Ranch
(TVR) in Tucson, AZ. TVR has been a huge part of our
Ripmaster/Dobson family adventures for decades. We
started going to the desert of Tucson, AZ in the early '80s.
It's amazing that even though I've lost my mom and dad,
my girls still have the opportunity to know their great
grandmother. Grandma Dobson is 98 years old as I write
this and living in Ann Arbor, MI. I'm a HUGE fan of my
Grandma Dobson.

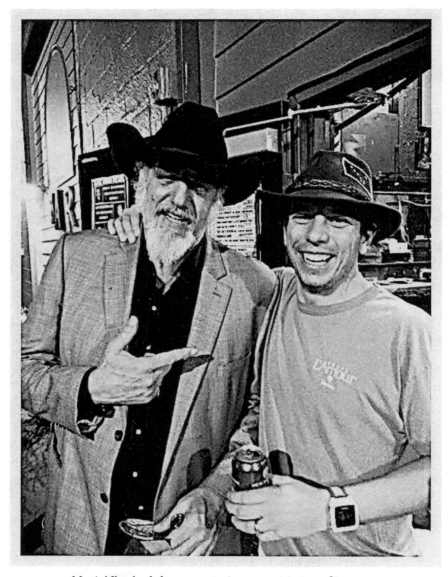

Music! I've had the opportunity to meet some of my very
favorite musicians. Here is a pictures of me and Ray Benson
from Asleep at the Wheel.

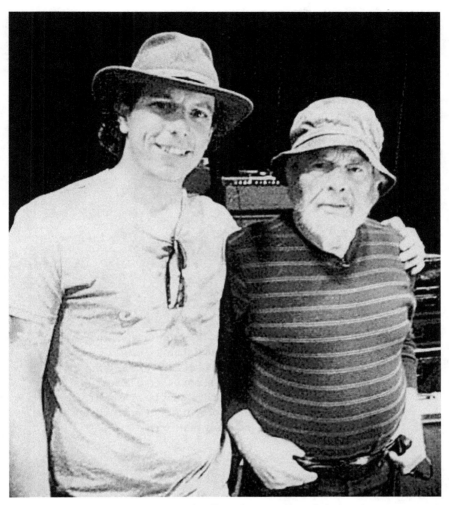

Meeting Merle Haggard will go down as one of the coolest moments of my entire life, and I'll never forget it because my dad passed away the very next day.

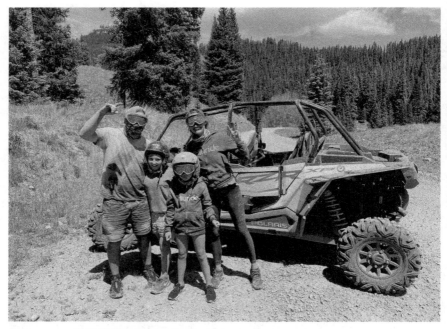

ADVENTURE! If I don't pass on my spirit of adventure to my girls then I will feel as if I failed them. Recently, we had a big family adventure riding a Polaris RZR in the Telluride backcountry. Even though I adore living in beautiful Asheville, NC, Telluride, CO will always be my spiritual home and my favorite small town in America. I think my girls feel the exact same way!